THE
BOOK OF
BURPEES

BE YOUR CLIENT'S FAVORITE **FITNESS**
TRAINER WITH THESE 100 BURPEE **EXERCISE**
VARIATIONS FOR YOUR **LESSON PLANS**!

SHANNON LUKEMAN HIROMASA
SHAIRA LUKEMAN

Legal and Copyright

Contents

Fitness and Exercise Disclaimer

Please review the following carefully

The purpose of this DISCLAIMER AND NOTICE is to make you conscious of the potential risks connected with activity in any exercise, physical fitness or training program. And to help you make an informed decision about whether you should participate in these activities.

You should understand that participating in any exercise or exercise program carries the possibility of physical injury. You should be in good physical condition and able to participate in the exercise. If you engage in this exercise or exercise program, you agree that you do so at your own risk, are voluntarily participating in these activities, and assume all risk of injury to yourself.

The information in this book is meant to supplement, not replace, proper personal or group fitness training. Like any sport involving speed, equipment, balance and environmental factors, performing burpees and other types of exercise shown here poses some inherent risk. The authors and publisher advise readers to take full responsibility for their safety and know their limits. Before practicing the skills described in this book and videos, be sure that your equipment is well maintained, and do not take risks beyond your level of experience, aptitude, training, and comfort level.

Injuries of all types can occur when participating in exercise, physical fitness and training programs, hence we strongly encourage all members to obtain a comprehensive physical examination by a licensed physician PRIOR to undertaking any exercise or training demonstrated in this book including all pictures and videos offered in this book of burpees. Such injuries include but are not limited to:

Bruising, cuts, and general soreness, Muscular and tendon injuries, Ligament and skeletal injuries, Fractured or broken bones, Concussions, Heart attack, OTHER

THE PUBLISHERS OF THIS BOOK EXPRESSLY DISCLAIMS LIABILITY FOR ALL DAMAGES AND ASSUMES NO LIABILITY OR RESPONSIBILITY FOR ANY LOSS, INJURY, OR DAMAGE SUFFERED BY ANY PERSON AS A RESULT OF THE USE, MISUSE, REFERENCE TO, RELIANCE ON, OR RESULTS OBTAINED FROM ANY INFORMATION, VIDEOS, AUDIO OR TRAINING MATERIALS MADE AVAILABLE IN THIS BOOK OR FROM INFORMATION OBTAINED AT LINKED SITES OR FEATURED AND/OR RECOMMENDED PRODUCTS.

Introduction

Use the Book of Burpees to create amazing and fun new lesson plans! Burpee variations are an excellent tool to enhance your fitness goals. Use them with your personal training clients and/or incorporate them into your group fitness classes. Use them to spice up your own personal workouts.

You will love the variations we include in this book! We give you 100+ done for you and easy to incorporate burpee variations into your workout sessions.

This book includes body weight burpees, burpees using various equipment, burpee regressions and modifications to safely address your clients' needs, and fitness challenges you can easily implement in any fitness format.

All the burpee variations include pictures, explanations and video links so that you can quickly view the burpee variation. This book is a must have for the caring and creative fitness enthusiast. We love burpees!

About the Authors

SHANNON:

Shannon is the best selling author of the book "Get Fit Done," creator of the hybrid kickboxing and cross training program Cross Kick, and the revolutionary new GET FIT DONE program. She is also an entrepreneur and co-owner of Colorado Krav Maga which has 5 locations across Colorado. She has been in the fitness and martial arts industry for over 30 years and counting. Her hobbies include kayaking, running, hiking, any outdoors activities as well as extreme races, Spartan races, Tough Mudders, and any race that is new and challenging! She enjoys seeing the transformation in her clients and how their lives improve. Her goal is to help everyone who needs it to just GET FIT DONE. She also LOVES BURPEES and all the glorious variations.

Shannon is the proud mother of 3 children who finally left the house and now she is an "empty nester." She is excited to put all that extra energy and time into her new program and books!

This book is exciting as it is co-produced with her own daughter, Shaira.

SHAIRA:

Shaira grew up as a competitive gymnast and fitness enthusiast. Her name is etched forever on the walls of her high school for beating out all the boys for the most push-ups! She loves obstacle racing, horses, dogs and horror movies.

She is a certified Krav Maga and fitness instructor as well as Get Fit Done Trainer. Locals call her the "Burpee Queen!"

Shaira loves helping others achieve their goals.

Shannon is available to teach Get Fit Done certifications (which include these burpees!) as well as speak about corporate wellness programs.

Go to: www.getfitdone.us for more information and/or to schedule a presentation or certification.

Brief History and Evolution of the Burpee

Before we bask in the awesomeness of 100 burpee variations – you might ask yourself: What is a burpee and where did it come from? Why the strange name?

The Burpee is named after its inventor, Dr. Royal H. Burpee. A Graduate of Columbia University with a degree in Physiology, he created the exercise during the 1930's as a rapid means to as-sess fitness levels. The United States Armed Services is credited with making the exercise popular when they used it to assess recruits' physical ability. The test evolved in a more demanding method to assess an individual's physical fitness capability during the WWII era. It was said Dr. Burpee didn't appreciate the way his exercise was applied at such a high intensity level. Well, times have certainly changed! (Source: https://en.wikipedia.org/w/index.php?title=Burpee_(exercise)&oldid=824975936)

Now you know! Thanks to Dr. Burpee for the exercise we love to hate the most. He had no idea it would evolve into the beast it is today.

The burpee is unforgiving and immediately tests a person's strength, endurance, core, coordination and agility.

The original burpee as invented by Dr. Burpee, consisted of only 4 moves known as the squat thrust. The moves were as follows:

1. Squat and place hands on the floor

2. Kick both feet back to a high plank

3. Return to the squat with hands on the floor

4. Stand up from the squat

The original "burpee" was of course a much simpler version than the burpee we know today. The full burpee version or regular burpee, as practiced today, includes a couple of more steps (all optional of course):

1. Squat and place hands on the floor

2. Kick both feet back to a high plank

3. Do a push-up

4. Return to high plank

5. Hop feet back to hands

6. Explode from the squat with hands on the floor into a vertical jump

So why do them?

Studies show that 15 minutes of high intensity interval training, such as burpee exercises, can burn more calories than an hour of jogging on a treadmill, helps boost your metabolism and post exercise calorie burn, and improves cardiovascular health, among other benefits! (source: http://www.healthfitnessrevolution.com/top-10-health-benefits-hiit-high-intensity-interval-training/).

The evolution of fitness in the last few decades means trainers are more creative in transferring their knowledge and helping clients achieve their goals. Now, it is common to do burpees in almost every fitness facility, and lately, to do burpee variations. The variations are simply additions and modifications using bodyweight or equipment to increase the variety of this whole-body exercise. Why not make something a little bit more exciting? The following burpee variations are some of the most creative hybrids of the burpees we could come up. Enjoy, and as always, be safe first and foremost.

You can find a link to a brief video of all of the burpees listed here by going to : http://www.getfitdone.us/book-of-burpees/

PART 1

BODYWEIGHT BURPEES

ALL OF THE burpees can be scaled to fit your clients' needs. Make sure you thoroughly assess your clients needs, fitness level and overall ability. Factors to keep in mind are medical impediments, age, flexibility and mobility, new to your program, prior or current injuries, temperature/environment, mood, etc.

In general, a good assessment before letting a client even attempt a burpee is: Can they hold a plank for 30 seconds? Holding a plank for at least 30 seconds is a good indicator if they can perform a burpee, which involves heavy use of the core. If they can't, or if they are just getting started in a fitness program, it is possible to modify almost all the burpees. Some of these regressions and modifications are listed in the burpee descriptions, some are not. We mixed it up to give you the most variety possible. Use common sense and understand your clients' ability and needs.

Following are some examples on scaling back any of the burpees where possible:

Add height. Have client place hands on an elevated surface, such as a plyo box or a bench.

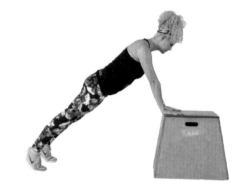

Get feet wider. This adds a more stable base during plank, push-ups, etc.

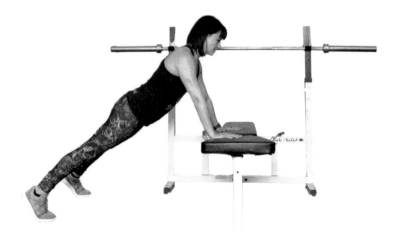

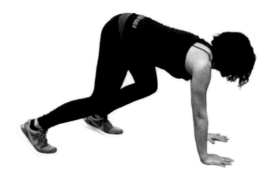

Walk it out. Have client inch-worm back and forth or step instead of jumping or hopping back and forth from plank.

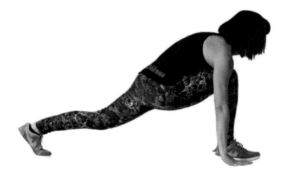

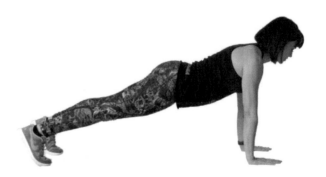

If the burpee calls for a push-up and the client is struggling, they can eliminate it altogether or perform the push-up off of the knees.

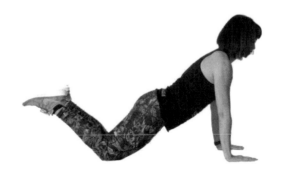

Keep it low impact. Especially for clients with any joint problems, eliminate the jump and have them simply return to stand or come up on toes. They can raise arms overhead or do a stepping jumping jack.

Be creative and modify according to your client's current ability. These basic modifications should help you formulate a workout ideal to your client.

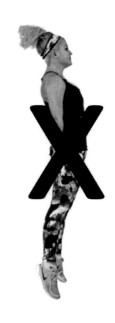

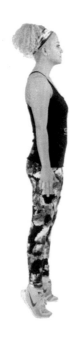

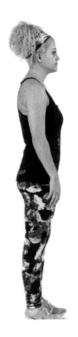

The basics: You might see a variation that indicates to "finish with a regular burpee". Sometimes there are pictures and other times there aren't. Here are the details on the regular burpee as widely used in the fitness world. We appreciate the most intense cross training styles out there as well, but in this book, we picked more of a squat version to floor version for most of the burpees, vs. a hip snap and kick back. No matter which style you prefer, encourage safety and form over reps.

We usually take a wider stance, with feet at or slightly outside of hands but also use the "blocking" method. Blocking means your feet are together and inside your hands in and out of the plank to the jump. It is more difficult and reserved for fit clients. We love them all.

THE BASIC, OR REGULAR OLD BURPEE

A Start in a standing position, feet approximately hip width apart, toes slightly outward.

B Shift weight back into heels, bend knees and start to squat.

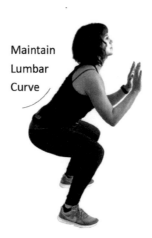

Maintain
Lumbar
Curve

C Hinge from hips as you place hands onto the ground, hands underneath shoulders, feet should be wider or right at the hands.

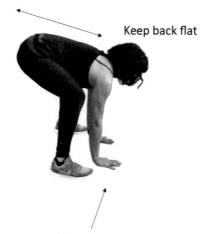

Keep back flat

Lower your hands to the
ground and spread fingers out
like stars

D Jump both feet back to a plank position.

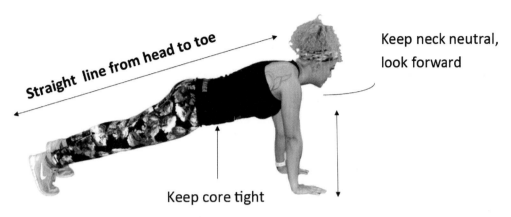

Straight line from head to toe

Keep neck neutral,
look forward

Keep core tight

Hands underneath shoulders,
push shoulders away from ears.

E Bend elbows and lower chest to ground for a push-up.

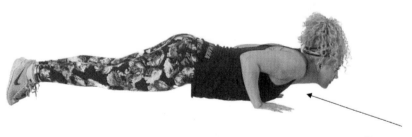

Keep elbows
close to body,
elbows back

F Complete push-up to return to plank position.

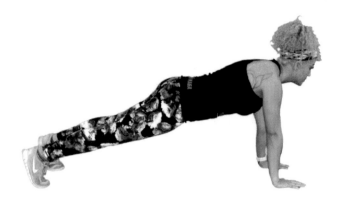

G Bend knees and jump both feet back towards hands, continue upwards motion into a jump to complete the regular burpee.

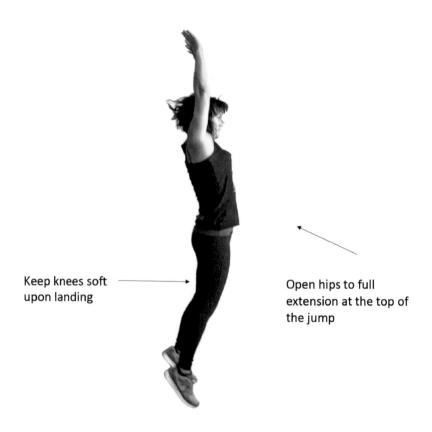

Keep knees soft upon landing

Open hips to full extension at the top of the jump

BURPEE VARIATION #1:

HALF BURPEE (WITH OR WITHOUT PUSH UP)

A Follow the beginning steps of a regular burpee to get into plank position.

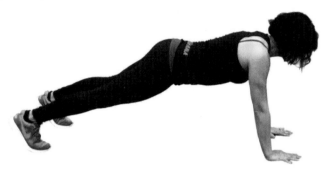

TRAINER'S TIP: Eliminating the push-up allows for a more intense cardio interval. Add the push-up for difficulty and a strength based burpee. Set a goal for # of reps before standing. For example, complete 4 half burpees before returning to standing position. Advanced clients can add a jump at the end of the set = CARDIO

B Bend knees and hop feet in towards hands and back out to plank, repeat that sequence for a set number of half burpee reps, or until you've had enough, then return to standing position to finish.

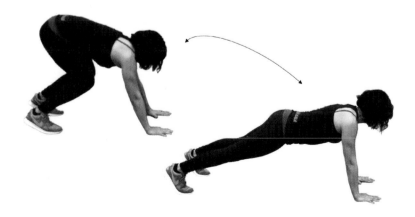

BURPEE VARIATION #2:

ONE LEGGED BURPEE

A Start in standing position, lift one leg up. Bend opposite leg as you shift hips back into a squat and reach for the ground.

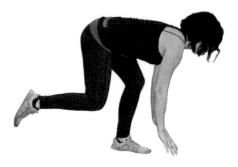

B Keeping that leg off the ground, plant hands and hop back on one foot to a single leg plank.

Don't overarch back
(no need to lift leg high)

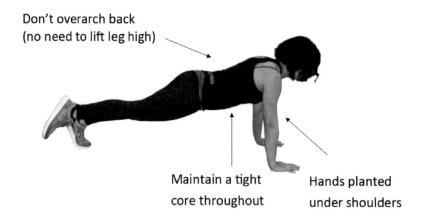

Maintain a tight
core throughout

Hands planted
under shoulders

Push-up.

Push-up

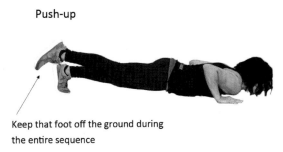

Keep that foot off the ground during
the entire sequence

D Straighten arms to plank, bend knees and hop back on one foot to hands and perform a single legged jump up.

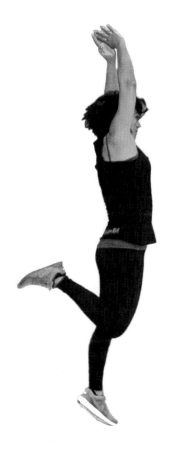

E After jump, put both feet down. Repeat sequence on other leg.

BURPEE VARIATION #3:

ONE ARM BURPEE

A From standing position, lift one arm out to side/front and the other one behind your back.

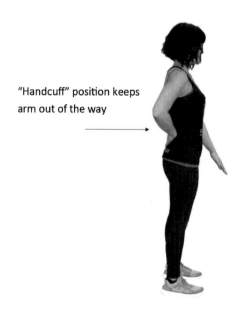

"Handcuff" position keeps arm out of the way

B Bend knees, squat and hop back to plank while staying on one hand.

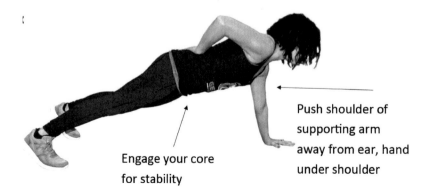

Engage your core for stability

Push shoulder of supporting arm away from ear, hand under shoulder

C Hop both feet back to squat (stay on single arm) and jump up.

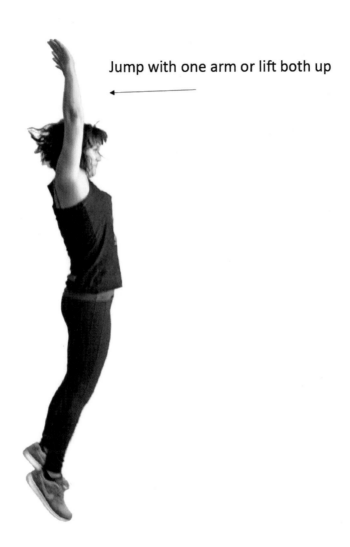

Jump with one arm or lift both up

D Reset stance, switch arms, and repeat one arm burpee sequence on the other side.

BURPEE VARIATION #4:

TUCK JUMP BURPEE

A Perform a regular burpee up to the push-up at the bottom.

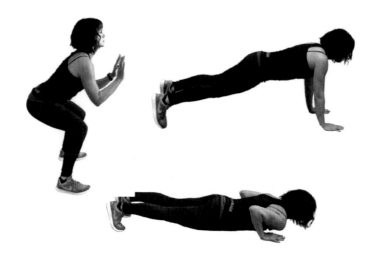

B Hop both feet back to hands, proceed to explode straight up as high as possible and tuck both knees under arms. Release knees quickly and land softly to stand.

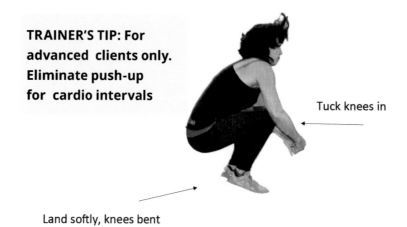

TRAINER'S TIP: For advanced clients only. Eliminate push-up for cardio intervals

Tuck knees in

Land softly, knees bent

BURPEE VARIATION #5:

STAR JUMP BURPEE

A Perform a regular burpee up to the push-up at the bottom.

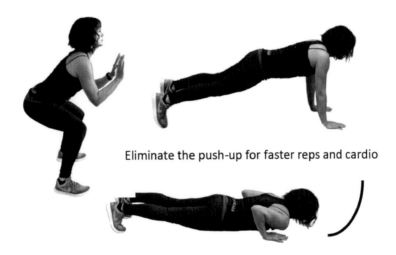

Eliminate the push-up for faster reps and cardio

B Hop both feet back to hands, proceed to explode straight up as high as possible while lifting arms and legs up and out to the sides in a "star" pattern. Bring feet together on the way down and land softly to stand.

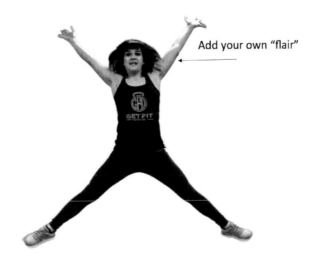

Add your own "flair"

BURPEE VARIATION #6:

JUMPING LUNGES BURPEE

A Perform a regular burpee up to the push-up at the bottom.

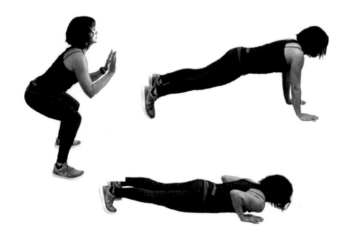

B Hop both feet back to hands and hop up, then step one leg back and jump lunge, switching legs 2-4 reps before bringing both feet back to standing.

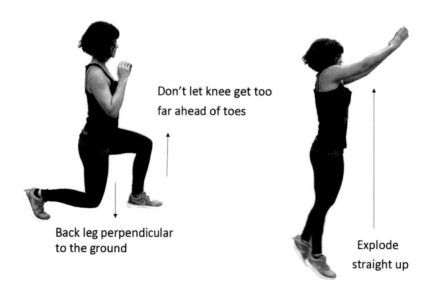

Don't let knee get too far ahead of toes

Back leg perpendicular to the ground

Explode straight up

B Continued -- Jump and switch legs each time for 2-4 reps before resetting to standing position.

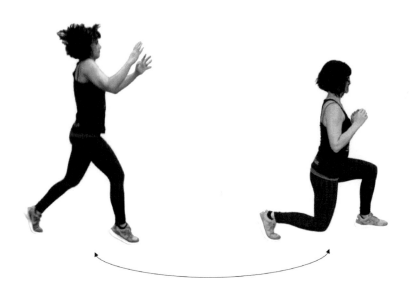

Jump and switch legs each time for 2-4 reps before resetting to standing position.

BURPEE VARIATION #7:

FROGGY BURPEE

A Perform a regular burpee up to the plank at the bottom.

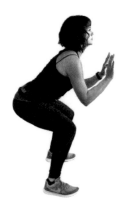
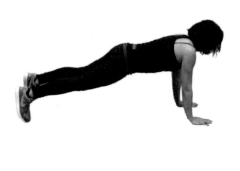

B Hop both feet to outside of hands and back to plank for two reps (froggy style)

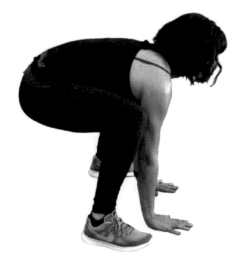

C Finish with a vertical jump.

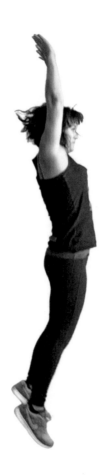

Make it easier with no jump at the top. Simply return to standing

BURPEE VARIATION #8:

CATERPILLAR BURPEE

A Start off by squatting, placing hands on floor, then walk both feet back to plank, taking small steps

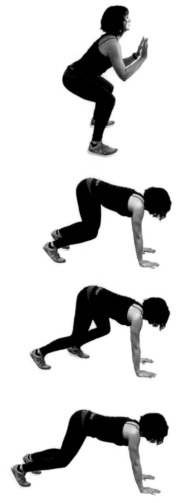

TRAINER'S TIP: Good variation for clients with injuries or for beginners. No impact

No push-up at the bottom. Trainers can add a push-up for another variation/difficulty.

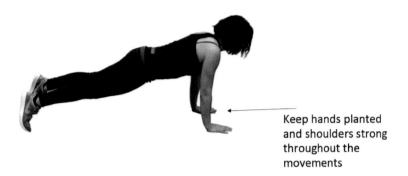

Keep hands planted
and shoulders strong
throughout the
movements

B Reverse the movement by walking feet back towards hands to starting position. Finish with a vertical jump.

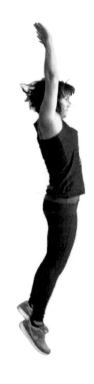

TRAINER'S TIP: make it easier and eliminate the jump

BURPEE VARIATION #9:

BROAD JUMP BURPEE

A Start standing, feet hip width apart. Jump forward as far as you can, land softly.

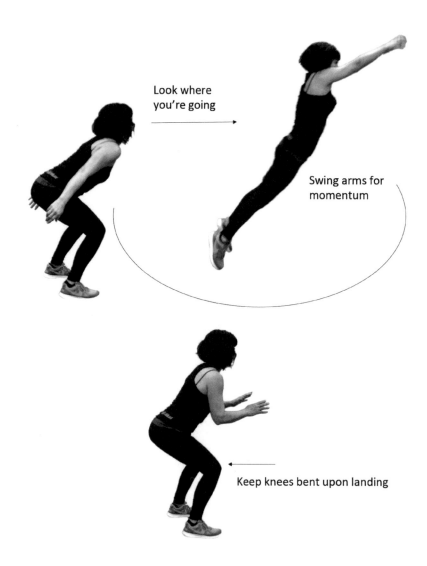

Look where you're going →

Swing arms for momentum

Keep knees bent upon landing

B Perform a 180-degree jump to face the side you came from.

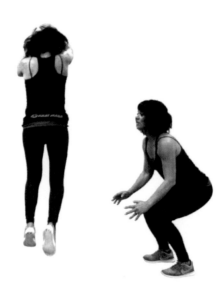

C Plank to push-up, bring feet back to hands and broad jump forward again instead of vertical. Land softly.

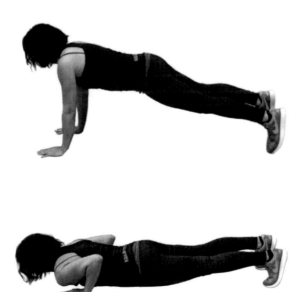

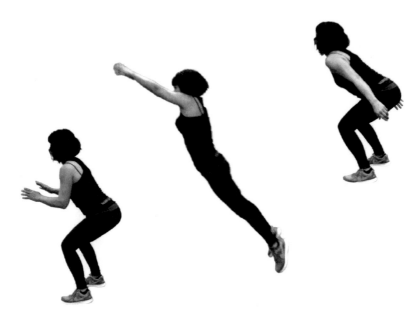

D 180 degree jump to end up in the same position you started.

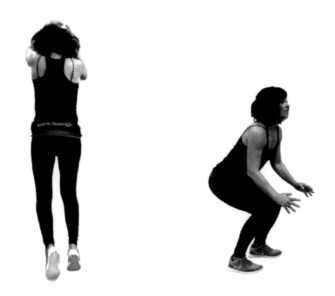

TRAINER'S TIP VARIATION: Have a goal in distance for the broad jump instead of turning around. For example, broad jump burpee between cones, for 300 meters, around the block, etc. depending on the class fitness level.

BURPEE VARIATION #10: SINGLE
LEG BROAD JUMP BURPEE

A Follow instructions for the Broad Jump Burpee, but perform all the moves on a single leg (can put foot down briefly after 180 degree jump.

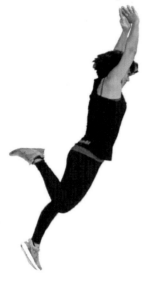

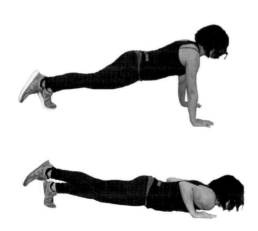

BURPEE VARIATION #11:

SIT THROUGH BURPEE

A Bend knees, hands to floor then hop feet back to plank and then hop feet forward to a "doggie" crouch .

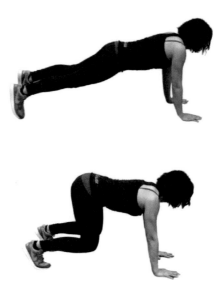

B Shift weight into your right hand, lift left arm up as you rotate torso and bring right leg underneath and through. Extend right leg all the way out to the side. Keep bottom to floor, while left leg is bent with weight in left heel.

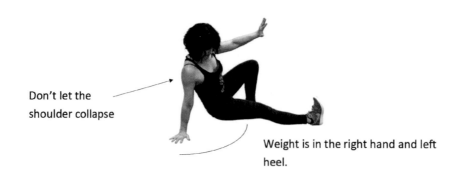

Don't let the shoulder collapse

Weight is in the right hand and left heel.

C Keeping weight on right hand/arm, reverse the motion by sliding right leg back through torso and placing left hand on the floor. Return to "doggie."

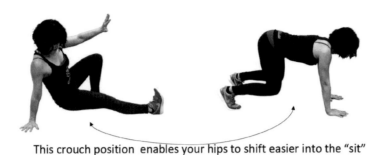

This crouch position enables your hips to shift easier into the "sit"

D Repeat sequence on other side, finish burpee with a vertical jump.

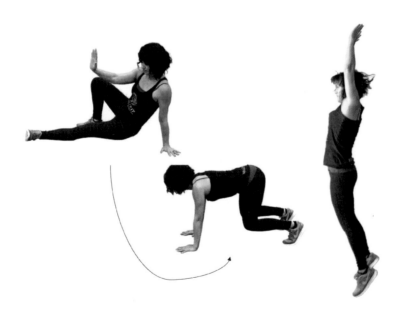

BURPEE VARIATION #12:

SPEED MOUNTAIN CLIMBER BURPEE

A Squat and bring hands to floor, hop back to plank. Quickly alternate bringing right knee in towards chest and then left knee towards chest in a rapid "climbing" motion. Alternate 4 times before returning to standing or vertical jump.

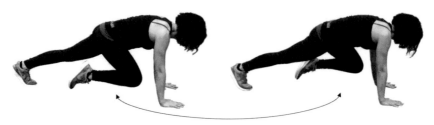

Switch knees rapidly

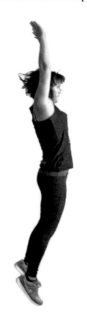

BURPEE VARIATION #13:

HIT THE DECK BURPEE

A Squat and hop feet back to plank, push-up, hop feet back to hands. Lift hands and rise up to a squat position.

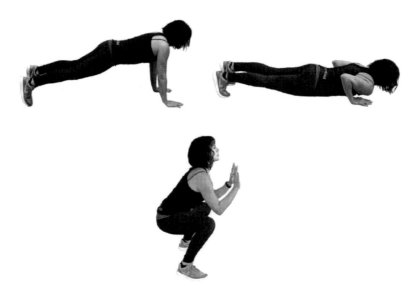

B From squat, shift weight back as you roll from bottom onto the back of shoulders .

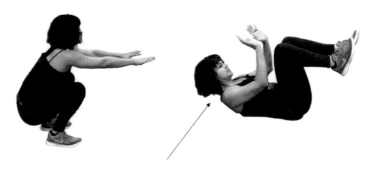

Don't roll onto head

C Reverse crunch, and use forward momentum to come out of the crunch and bring both feet back to the floor. Continue to push through heels and up into a squat, push off legs and jump straight up.

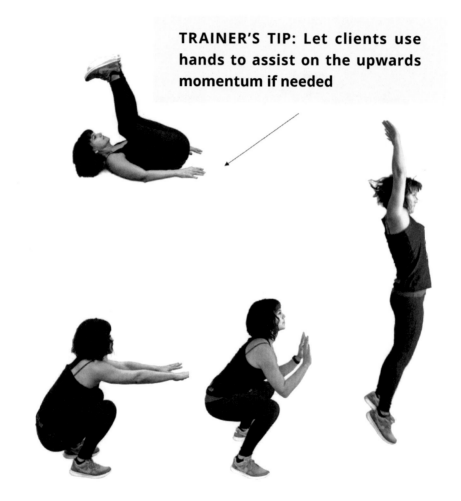

TRAINER'S TIP: Let clients use hands to assist on the upwards momentum if needed

BURPEE VARIATION
#14: TWISTED BURPEE

A From standing position, squat and place both hands on the floor.

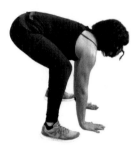

B Rotate your torso as you hop both feet back onto one side, feet stacked into a "twisted" high plank.

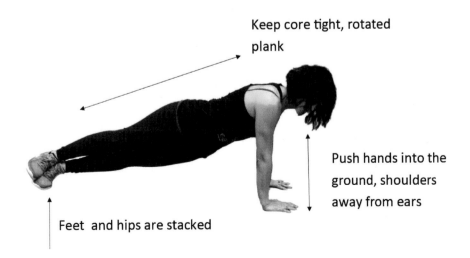

Keep core tight, rotated plank

Push hands into the ground, shoulders away from ears

Feet and hips are stacked

C From "twisted" plank, look towards open side and perform one push-up.

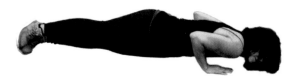

TRAINER'S TIP: Eliminate the push-up if your client has a weak core. Focus on core stability. Stagger one foot in front of the other (toes to floor) for assisted balance

D Hop both feet back towards hands, finish the burpee with a vertical jump. Repeat twisted burpee on the other side.

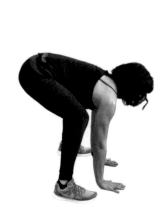

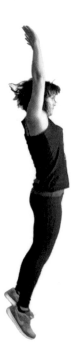

BURPEE VARIATION #15:

T PUSH-UP BURPEE

A Squat and hop both feet back to plank and push-up.

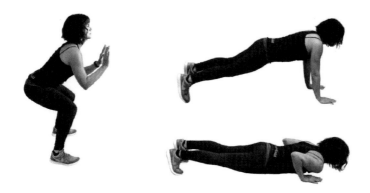

B At the top of the push-up, rotate torso as you lift one arm perpendicular into a "T" position.

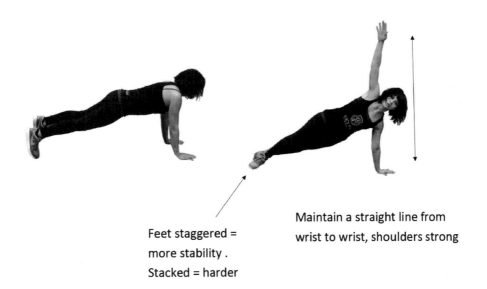

Feet staggered = more stability .
Stacked = harder

Maintain a straight line from wrist to wrist, shoulders strong

C Return to plank and push-up. Repeat "T" rotation on the other side..

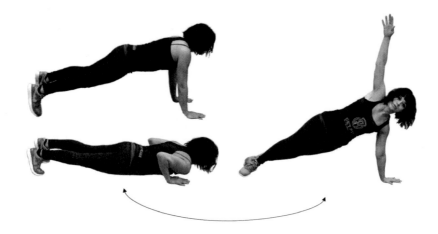

D Return to plank, hop feet back to hands, finish with a vertical jump.

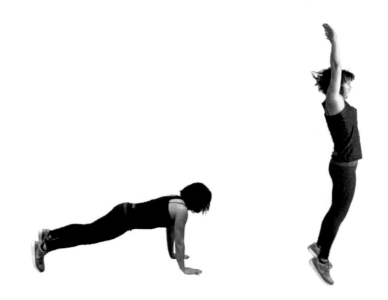

TRAINER'S TIP: Client can bring one knee down for added stability. Eliminate the push-ups in between torso rotation for an easier version

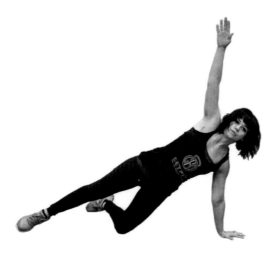

BURPEE VARIATION #16:

GRASSHOPPER BURPEES

A Squat, bring hands to floor and hop feet back to plank.

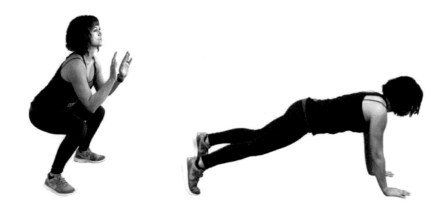

B Quickly hop right foot to left wrist and back, then rapidly repeat with left foot to right wrist and back. Complete 2 full sets (4 counts).

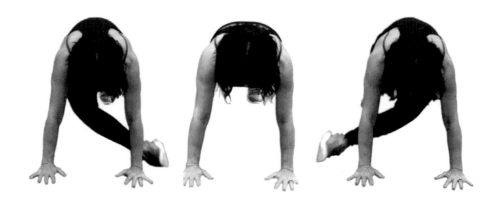

C Return to plank, hop feet back to hands and do a vertical jump.

No push-up

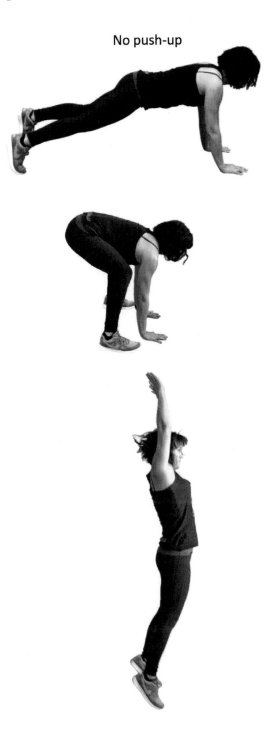

BURPEE VARIATION #17:

SPIDEY BURPEE

A Squat, bring hands to floor and hop feet back to plank.

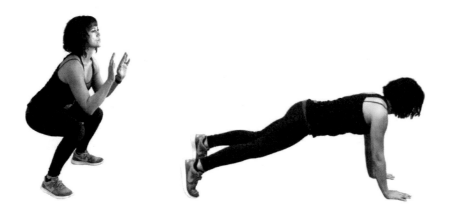

B Do a "spiderman" push-up by bringing one knee to same side elbow at the bottom of the push-up. Plank. Repeat "spiderman" push-up on other side.

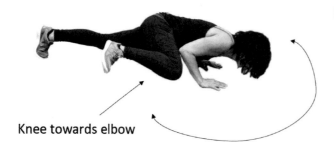

Repeat once on each side

Knee towards elbow

C Return to plank, hop hands to feet and perform a vertical jump.

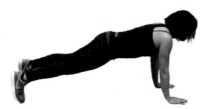

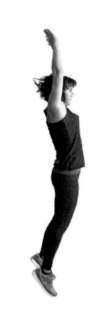

BURPEE VARIATION #18:

POWER UP BURPEE

A Squat, bring hands to floor, hop back to plank. Lower belly to ground. Both feet come up (superman) as both hands come up (palms down) and then back down. Press hands into the floor and back to plank.

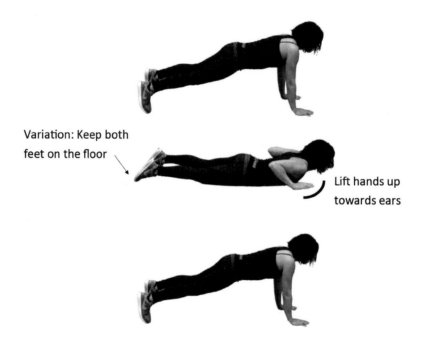

Variation: Keep both feet on the floor

Lift hands up towards ears

B Hop both feet back to hands and perform a vertical jump.

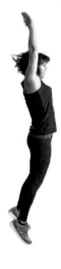

BURPEE VARIATION #19:

ELEVATOR BURPEE

A Squat, bring hands to floor and hop back to plank. Lower onto forearms one arm at a time into a low plank (hover), then back up into a high plank one arm at a time.

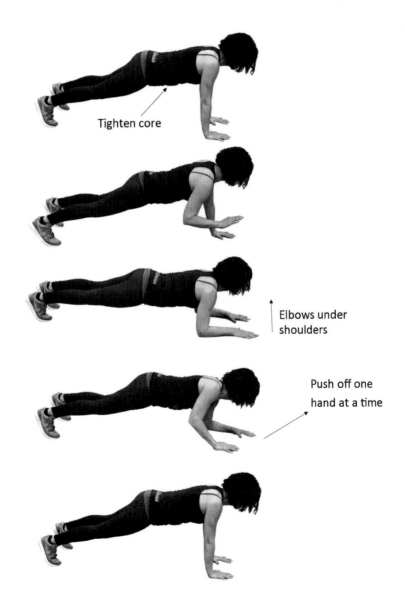

Tighten core

Elbows under shoulders

Push off one hand at a time

B From plank, hop feet back to hands and perform a vertical jump.

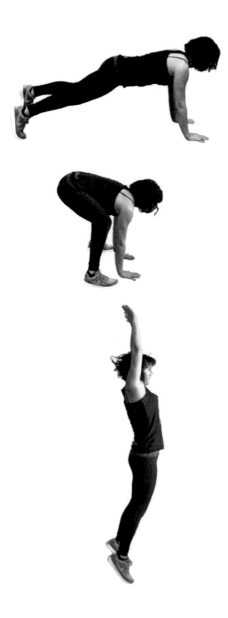

BURPEE VARIATION #20:

PLANK JACK BURPEE

A Squat, bring hands to floor and hop feet back to plank.

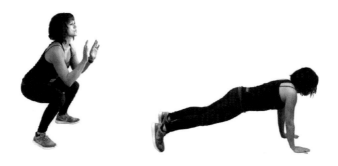

B From plank, open and close feet in a "jumping jack" motion. Feet open wide than narrow.

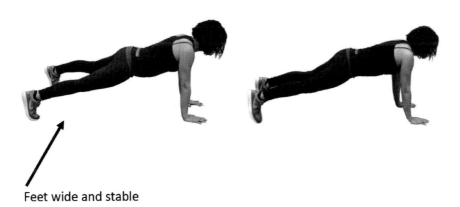

Feet wide and stable

C Hop both feet back to hands and jump up.

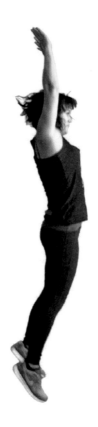

TRAINER'S TIP: Add more plank jacks to increase cardio and difficulty. Add a push-up as legs open for added difficulty.

BURPEE VARIATION #21:

DIRTY DOUBLE JACK BURPEE

A Start from standing position, hands by side. Jump up as high as possible while lifting arms and legs up and out to the sides in a "star" pattern. Bring feet together on the way down and land softly.

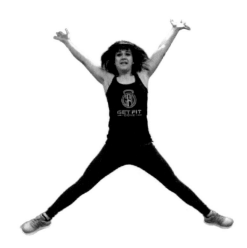

B Squat, bring hands to floor and hop both feet back to plank.

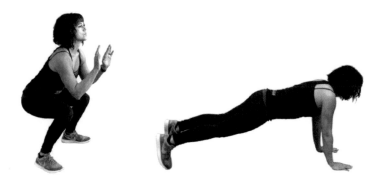

C From plank, open and close feet in a "jumping jack" motion. Feet open wide than narrow.

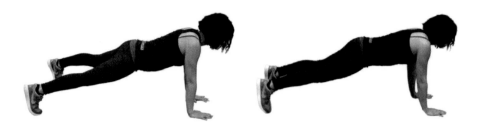

D Hop both feet back to hands, and explode up into another star jump.

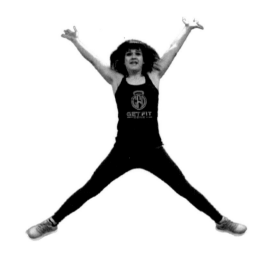

BURPEE VARIATION #22:

ALTERNATING ARM RAISE BURPEE

A Squat, bring hands to floor and hop both feet back to plank.

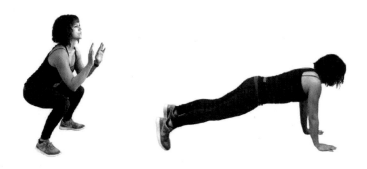

B From plank, lower into a push-up. As you straighten arms back to plank, lift one arm up in front of you (shoulder height) and back down to plank, then push-up again and lift the other arm up to shoulder height and back to plank.

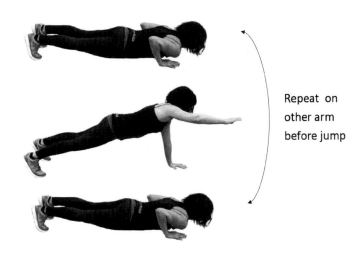

Repeat on other arm before jump

C Hop both feet back to hands and jump straight up.

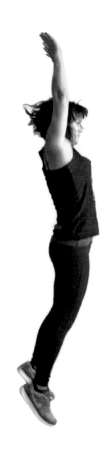

TRAINER'S TIP: Eliminate the push-ups in between arm raises to make it easier for client.

BURPEE VARIATION #23:

SHOULDER TAP BURPEE

A Squat, bring hands to floor and hop both feet back to plank and push-up.

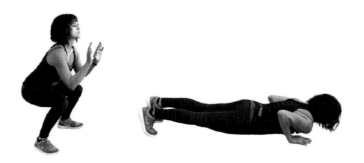

B From plank, lower into a push-up. As you straighten arms back to plank, lift one hand up and lightly tap opposite shoulder. Return to plank and repeat push-up. Repeat shoulder tap with opposite hand. Return to plank.

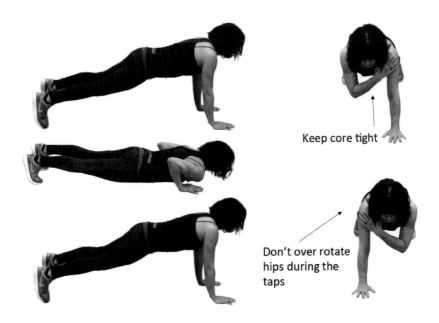

Keep core tight

Don't over rotate hips during the taps

C Hop both feet back to hands and jump straight up.

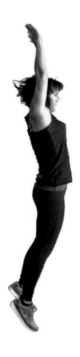

TRAINER'S TIP: Keep feet wider at the bottom of the plank to increase stability during the shoulder taps.

Eliminate the push-ups in between shoulder taps to make this exercise easier.

BURPEE VARIATION #24:

INCH WORM BURPEE

A Squat and lower hands in front of feet. Walk hands forward while feet stay in place until body is in a plank position. Reverse the motion by walking hands back towards feet. Stand up and finish with a vertical jump.

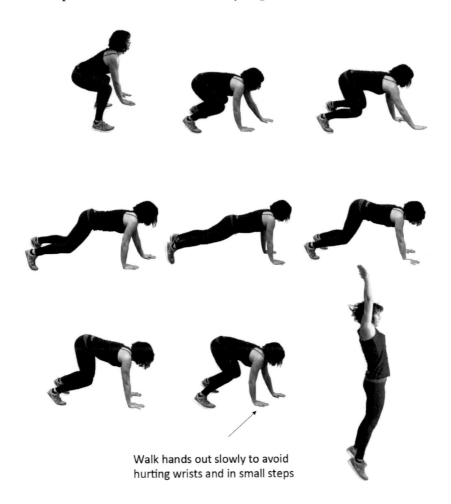

Walk hands out slowly to avoid hurting wrists and in small steps

BURPEE VARIATION #25:

ZEN BURPEE CORE BURNER (INSPIRED BY YOGA)

A Squat, bring hands to floor and hop both feet back to plank.

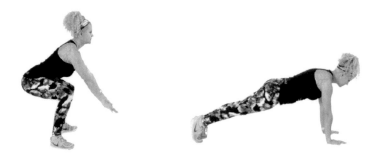

B Push-up and come back to plank. Lift one leg off the ground and bend knee in towards nose and back out.

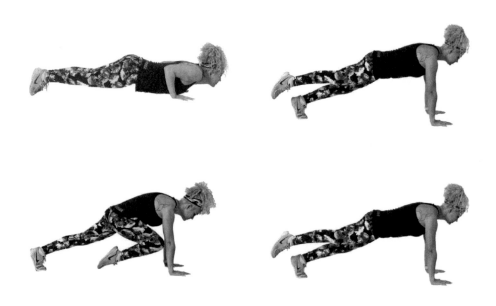

C Keeping the same leg off the ground, bend knee in towards opposite elbow and back out.

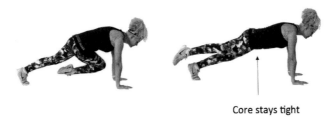

Core stays tight

D Keeping the same leg off the ground, bend knee in again towards the outside of the same side elbow and back out

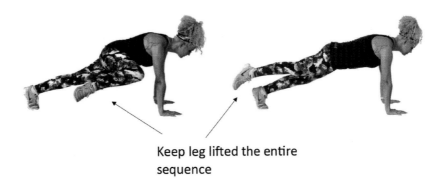

Keep leg lifted the entire sequence

E Lower leg back into plank, hop both feet back towards hands and jump up. Repeat sequence on other leg.

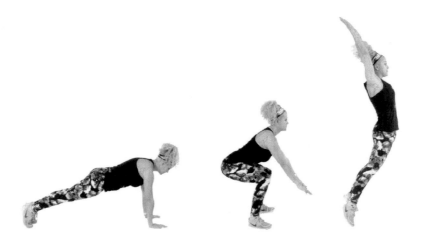

BURPEE VARIATION #26:

LATERAL KICK BURPEE

A Squat, bring hands to floor and hop both feet back to plank.

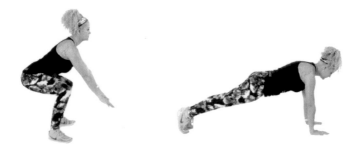

B Push-up at the same time you kick one leg out to the side then back to plank. Push-up again as you kick the other leg out to the side and back to plank.

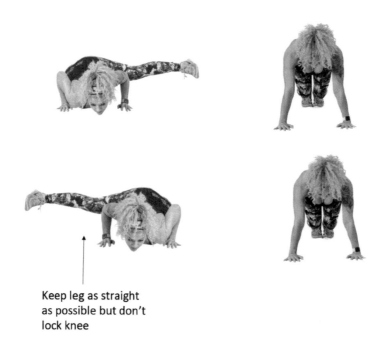

Keep leg as straight as possible but don't lock knee

C Hop both feet back to hands and finish with a vertical jump.

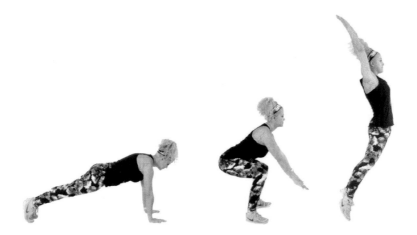

TRAINER'S TIP: Eliminate the push-up during the leg kick to make it easier.

BURPEE VARIATION #27:

DONKEY KICKS BURPEE

A Squat, bring hands to floor and hop both feet back to plank.

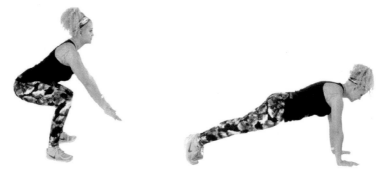

B Push-up, hop feet in, then explosively kick both feet up at the same time, heels towards the ceiling, land and repeat for 2 reps.

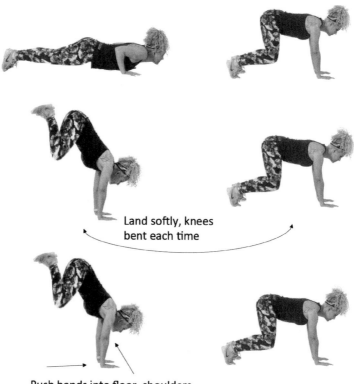

Land softly, knees bent each time

Push hands into floor, shoulders away from ears.

C Bring feet back to hands and finish with a vertical jump.

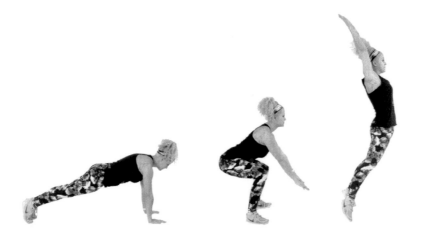

TRAINER'S TIP: This exercise is for advanced clients only.

BURPEE VARIATION #28:

SPRAWL BURPEE

A Do a regular burpee all the way through including the jump.

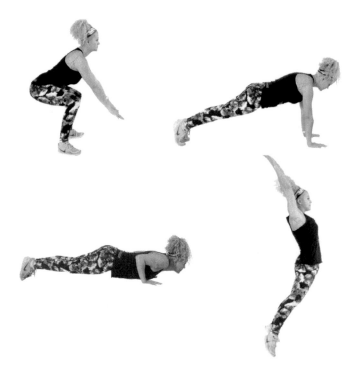

B After you land, bring both hands down to the floor in front of you, scoot both legs backward, hips towards floor and head up.

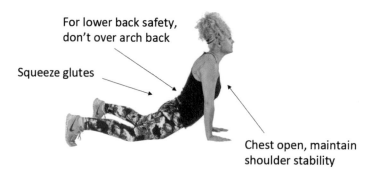

For lower back safety, don't over arch back

Squeeze glutes

Chest open, maintain shoulder stability

Hop both feet back to hands and jump straight up.

There is no push up after the sprawl.

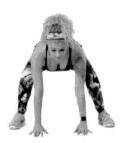

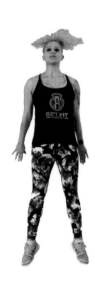

TRAINER'S TIP: Not recommended for clients with lower back problems who may over arch the back during the sprawl. Add more sprawls for increased difficulty before finish.

BURPEE VARIATION #29:

HI KNEES BURPEE

A Alternate high knees to hands for 4 reps.

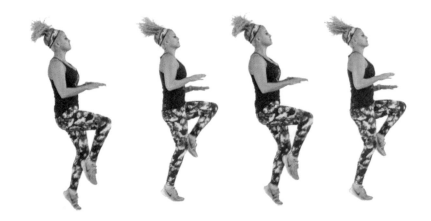

B Do a regular burpee all the way through including the jump.

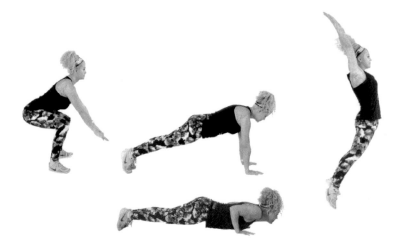

TRAINER'S TIP: Eliminate the push-up and repeat the burpee sequence for higher reps to increase cardio challenge

BURPEE VARIATION #30:

LATERAL JUMP BURPEE

A Squat, hands to floor, hop both feet back to plank and do a push-up. Come back to plank position.

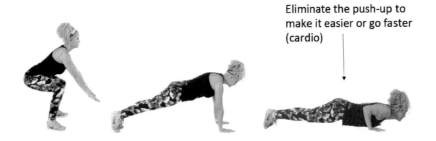

Eliminate the push-up to make it easier or go faster (cardio)

TRAINER'S TIP: A variation is to start with the lateral jump

B From plank, hop both feet to hands and jump laterally to one side. Land softly. Complete another regular burpee, jumping laterally instead of vertically. Repeat as many times as you want.

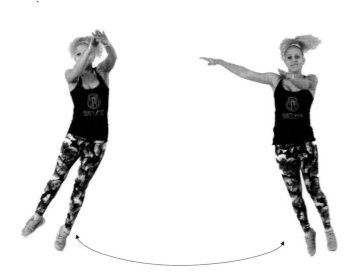

Jump laterally instead of vertically. Use arms for momentum. Knees soft upon landing.

BURPEE VARIATION #31: SLURPEE BURPEE

A Start by lying down on your back with both arms extended behind head, arms and legs straight. Using momentum, crunch up from sitting to standing position and jump straight up.

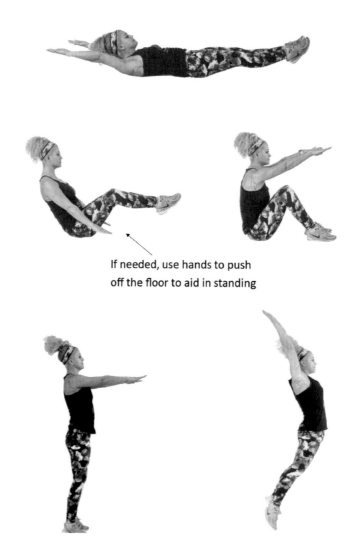

If needed, use hands to push off the floor to aid in standing

B Reverse the motion by sitting back down and returning to original position on back, face up, arms extended behind back and legs extended in front.

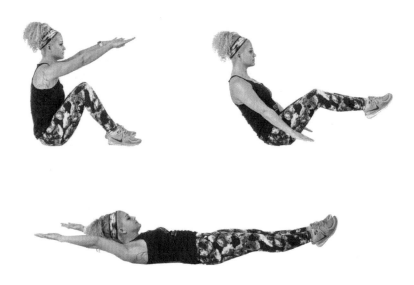

TRAINER'S TIP: This exercise is for advanced clients only. You can also perform this burpee starting from a standing position.

BURPEE VARIATION #32:

SUCK IT UP BURPEE

A Do a regular burpee all the way through including the jump.

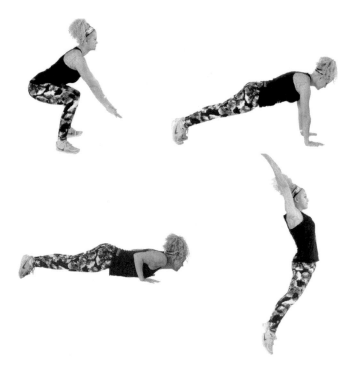

B After the jump, land softly. Bend knees and sit down, using momentum and rolling backwards onto shoulders and into a reverse crunch.

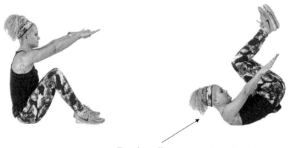

Don't roll onto neck or head

C Roll forward using momentum to get back to standing position, jump straight up into a tuck jump. Land softly.

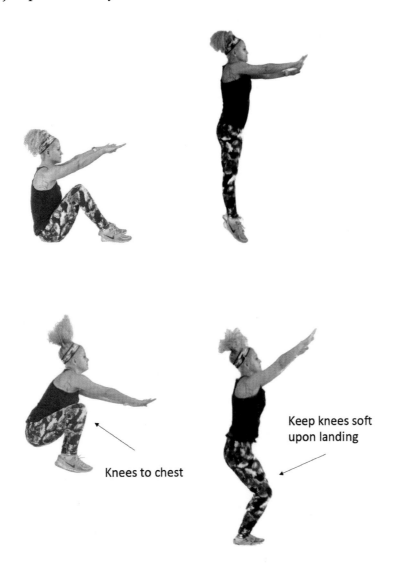

Knees to chest

Keep knees soft upon landing

TRAINER'S TIP: This exercise is for advanced clients only. You can eliminate the tuck jump to make it easier.

BURPEE VARIATION #33:

DIVEBOMBER BURPEE

A Squat, hands to floor and hop feet back to plank. Lift tailbone up and hips back, heels towards the floor in an inverted "V."

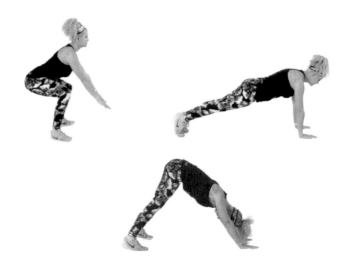

B Bend elbows and "scoop" body forward and up, hips to floor, looking up. Reverse the motion and "scoop" backwards to an inverted "V."

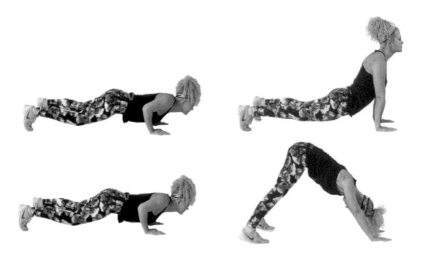

C Hop feet back to hands and jump straight up.

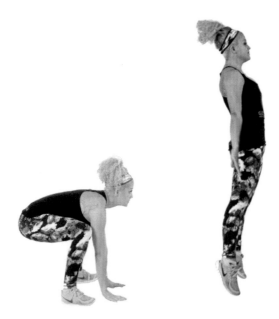

BURPEE VARIATION #34:

NINJA BURPEE

A Start on knees and lean slightly back. Stay low as you push off feet, bring knees up and land in a squat, feet underneath knees.

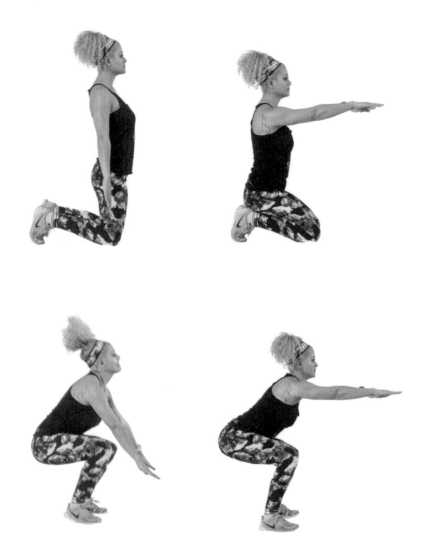

B From squat, bring hands back down to floor, hop both feet back to plank and push-up. Hop both feet back to hands and finish with a vertical jump.

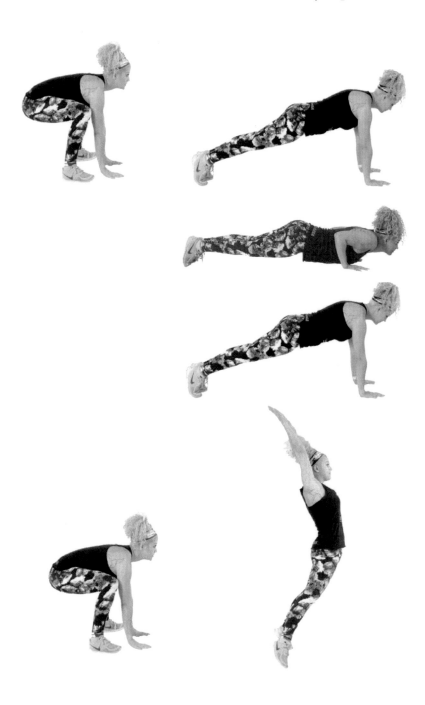

BURPEE VARIATION #35:

CROW POSE BURPEE

A Do a burpee all the way through the push-up.

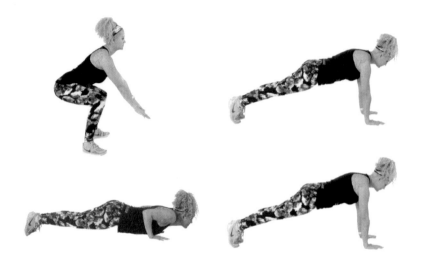

B Hop both feet towards hands. Bend elbows and lift one knee and place over same side elbow, lifting foot off the ground. Repeat with the other knee. Balance on both hands. Hold for 2-4 seconds. Put feet down and hop up to a vertical jump.

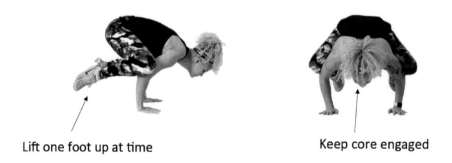

Lift one foot up at time

Keep core engaged

TRAINER'S TIP: Make it easier by keeping one foot on the ground while the other one is up.

BURPEE VARIATION #36:

YOGA BURPEE

A Squat, hands to floor and hop feet back to plank. Bend elbows and "scoop" body into upward facing dog, hip and shins off the floor.

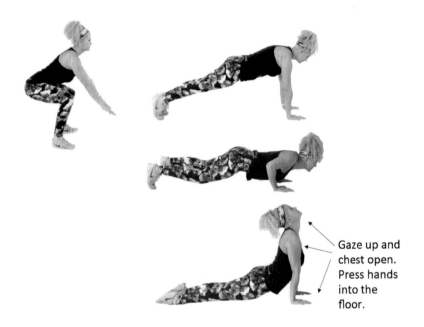

Gaze up and chest open. Press hands into the floor.

B Lift tailbone up and shift hips back, pressing heels towards the floor into downwards facing dog pose (inverted "V").

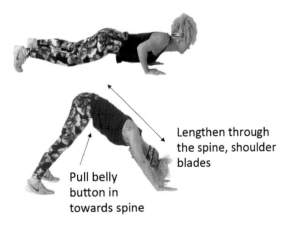

Lengthen through the spine, shoulder blades

Pull belly button in towards spine

C Hop both feet back to hands and jump straight up.

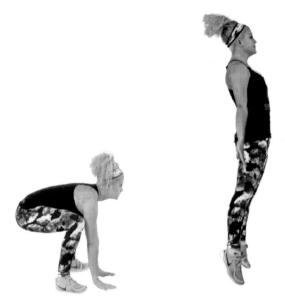

TRAINER'S TIP: Less flexible clients may keep heels off the floor in downward facing dog and focus on lengthening through the spine.

BURPEE VARIATION #37:

SLALOM BURPEE

A Bend knees and bring hands to floor. Jump both feet back and keep them together as you hop to one side and then back to the center and then to the other side and back to the center.

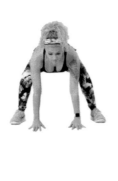

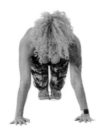

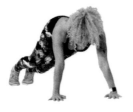

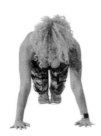

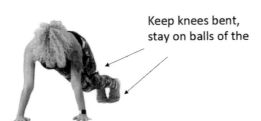

Keep knees bent, stay on balls of the

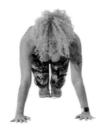

B Hop both feet back to hands and finish with a vertical jump.

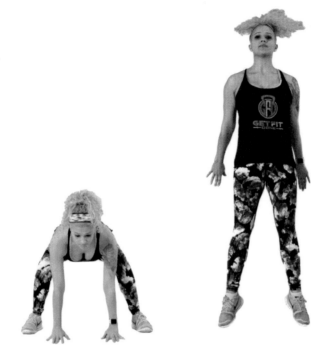

No push-ups

BURPEE VARIATION #38:

LUNGE & KICK BURPEE

A Step into a reverse lunge, then perform a front kick with the leg that stepped back into the lunge. Bringing kicking leg back down next to the other foot.

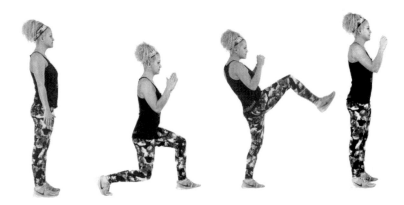

B After setting leg down, complete a regular burpee through the jump. Repeat lunge and kick on the other leg and end with a regular burpee.

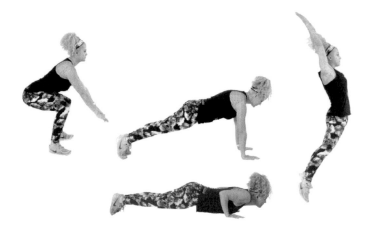

BURPEE VARIATION #39:

PLYOMETRIC PUSH-UP BURPEE

A Squat down, hands to floor and hop both feet back to plank. Bend elbows and push off hands explosively to get enough height where hands leave the ground. Land softly.

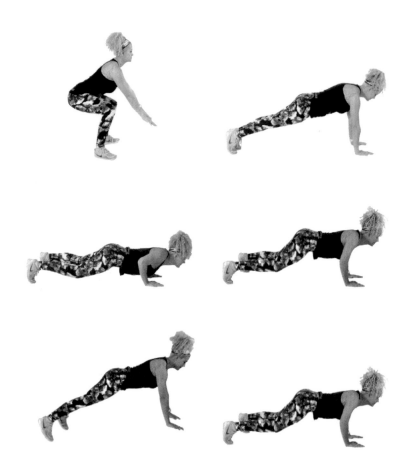

B Hop both feet back to hands and finish with a vertical jump.

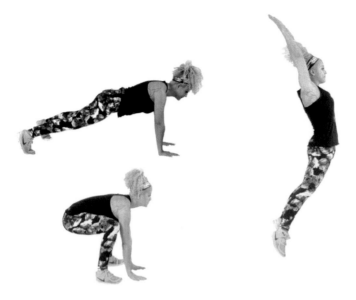

TRAINER'S TIP: For advanced clients only. Avoid faceplants. Variation for added difficulty: Clap hands together after exploding up and landing (shown in video)

BURPEE VARIATION #40:

PISTOL BURPEE

A Squat, bring hands to floor and hop feet back to plank. Do a push-up.

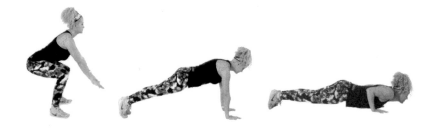

B After the push-up, hop both feet back to hands. Lift hands up and stay in a deep squat. Extend one leg in front of body so that you are in a pistol squat. Hold briefly then bring leg back and extend other leg to pistol squat. Jump up to finish the burpee.

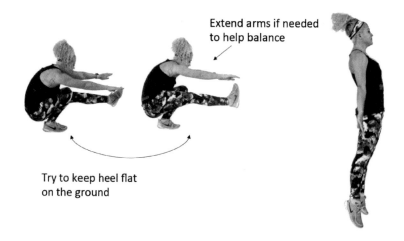

Extend arms if needed to help balance

Try to keep heel flat on the ground

TRAINER'S TIP: This exercise is for advanced and injury free clients.

BURPEE VARIATION #41:

SNOWBOARD STYLE BURPEE

A Jump and switch rapidly from side to side. Jump and squat diagonally while reaching hand towards the floor. Alternate sides for 3 snowboard style jumps. Stay low after last touch and go into a diagonal plank. Hop both feet back to hands, stay low and repeat sequence of 3 jump/touches and plank. End with a jump on the side you completed the last plank.

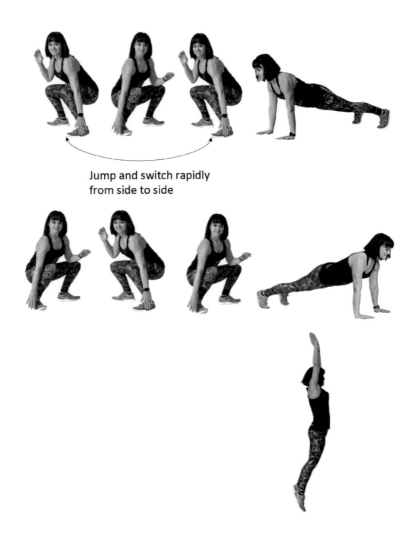

Jump and switch rapidly
from side to side

BURPEE VARIATION #42:

LOW SQUAT BURPEE

A Start and end the burpee from a low squat. Squat to plank, push-up and back. No jump. This is purely a leg burner.

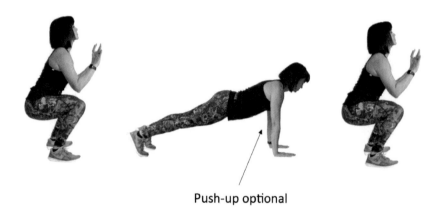

Push-up optional

Variation: Add a jump after a set amount of reps as a finisher. Example 4 low squat burpees and a vertical jump = one burpee

BURPEE VARIATION #43:

BULLDOG BURPEE

A Bend knees, bring hands to floor and jump back on all fours, knees stay bent and off the ground. Hop both feet back to hands then jump up to finish the burpee.

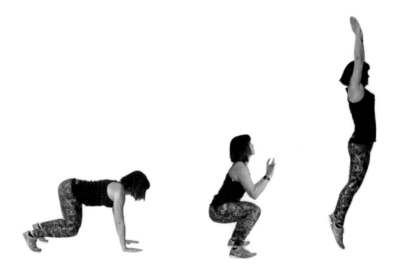

BURPEE VARIATION #44:

CORN ON THE COB BURPEE

A Squat and bring hands to floor. Hop feet back to plank. Bend elbows so that your face is hovering off of the floor. Imagine you are eating corn on the cob and stay low as you move from one side to the other.

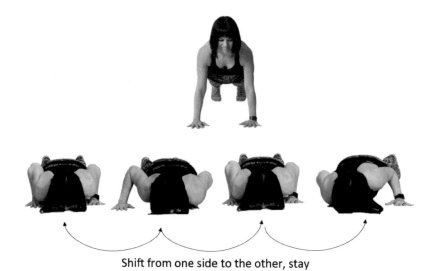

Shift from one side to the other, stay

B Return to center, push back up to plank, hop both feet to hands and jump up.

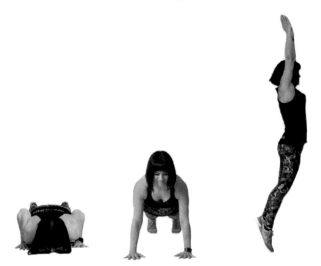

BURPEE VARIATION #45:

HIP DIP BURPEE

A Squat, hands to floor and hop back to plank. Shift onto forearms and hands, then twist and "tap" one side of the hips to floor. Return to center, then twist and "tap" other side of the hips to the floor.

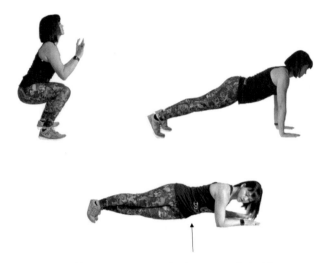

Focus on core control as you rotate hips

B Return to plank, hop both feet back to hands then jump up.

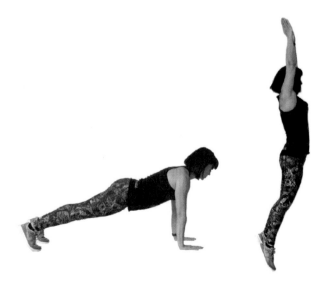

BURPEE VARIATION #46:

SKATER BURPEE

A Swing arms and skate to the side, keeping the opposite leg off of the floor. Hop back into a one legged plank, then hop back up on both feet. Jump straight up. Repeat to the other side.

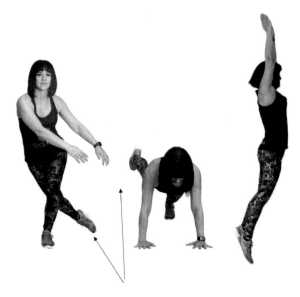

Keep that foot off the floor through the plank

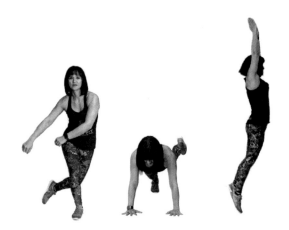

BURPEE VARIATION #47:

BIRD DOG BURPEE

A Squat, bring hands to floor and hop both feet back to plank.

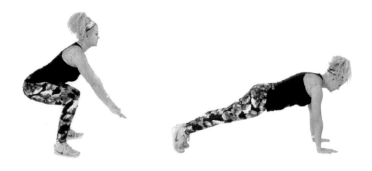

B Lift one arm straight in front of you at the same time you lift the opposite leg straight up behind you. Return to plank and repeat on the opposite side. Hop both feet to hands and jump up.

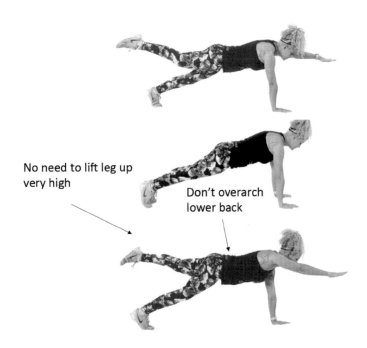

No need to lift leg up very high

Don't overarch lower back

C Hop both feet back to hands and jump up.

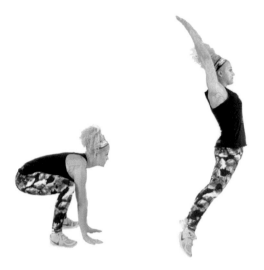

TRAINER'S TIP: This is the advanced version. Make it easier by going from plank to all fours, then lifting arm/leg from that position.

VARIATION: Add a crunch after leg and arm extension by bending knee of extended leg and crunching in towards elbow of extended arm.

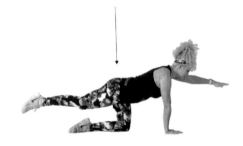

BURPEE VARIATION #48:

DOUBLE FRONT KICK BURPEE

A Squat, bring hands to floor and hop both feet back to plank and back to hands.

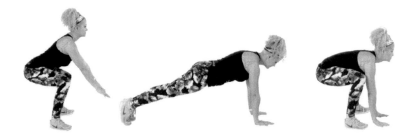

B Jump up and complete 2 front kicks, alternating legs.

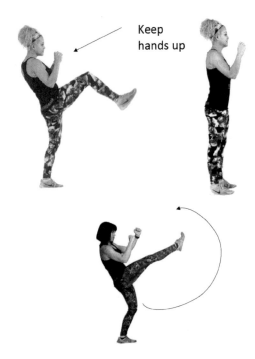

Keep hands up

TRAINER'S TIP: Flexible clients can kick higher and straighten leg more

BURPEE VARIATION #49:

HIPPITY HOP BURPEE

A Lower into a squat. Stay in a low squat and hop forward 3 times.

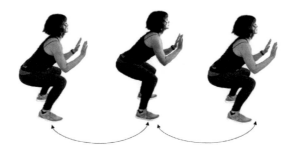

B After 3 hops, 180 degree jump to turn around and face opposite direction.

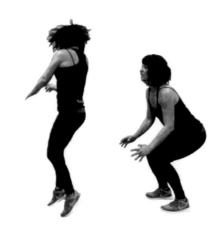

C Drop down, push-up and jump up.

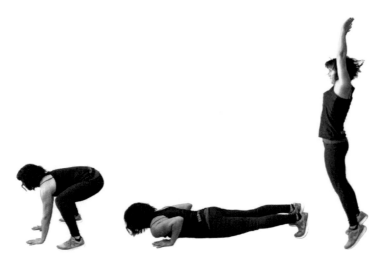

D Hop forward in a low squat 3 more times to end the burpee.

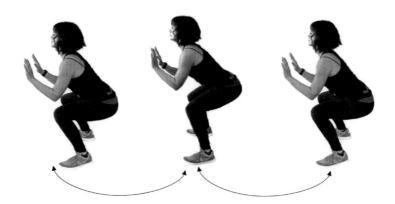

TRAINER'S TIP: Not recommended for clients with knee or impact issues.

Variation: Make it a leap frog by squatting low and touching the ground, or a prison walk burpee by bringing hands behind head.

BURPEE VARIATION #50:

CROUCHING TIGER BURPEE

A Squat, bring hands to floor and hop both feet back to plank.

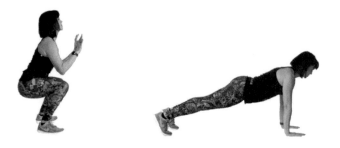

B Bend elbows, stay down and low. Move forward while pushing off toes and hands, elbows up. Next, move backwards while bringing elbows and forearms flat towards the floor.

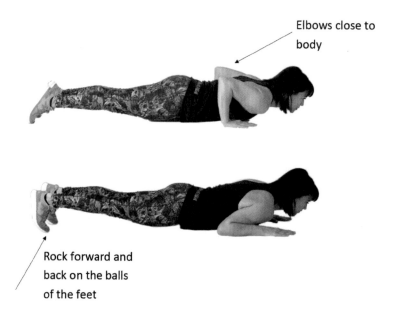

Elbows close to body

Rock forward and back on the balls of the feet

C Center, straighten arms back to plank, hop feet to hands and jump straight up to finish the burpee.

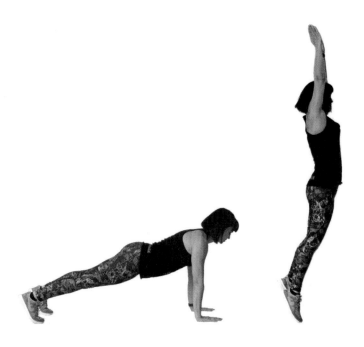

BURPEE VARIATION #51:

PLANK EXTENSION BURPEE

A Squat, bring hands to floor and hop both feet back to plank.

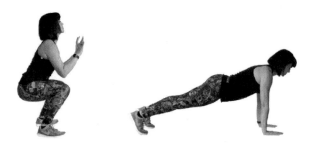

B Taking little steps, walk feet back while keeping hands in place. Extend through the plank as far as you can and then walk feet back to high plank. Finish with a vertical jump.

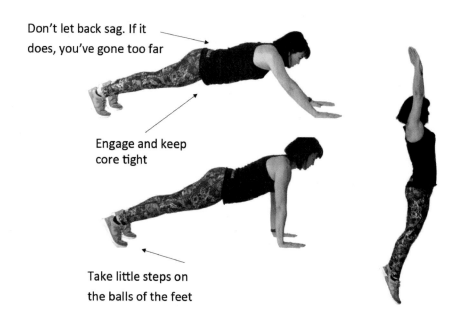

Don't let back sag. If it does, you've gone too far

Engage and keep core tight

Take little steps on the balls of the feet

BURPEE VARIATION #52:

SINGLE ARM SCAPULAR PUSH-UP BURPEE

A Squat, bring hands to floor and hop both feet back to plank.

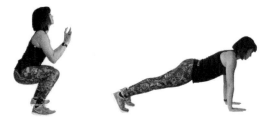

B Lift one hand up and place on opposite shoulder. Rotate elbow in towards elbow of planted arm. Return to plank, hop both feet to hands and jump up. Repeat sequence on opposite side. End with the vertical jump.

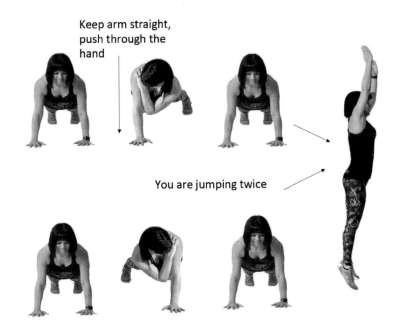

BURPEE VARIATION #53:

WAVING SUPERMAN BURPEE

A Squat, bring hands to floor and hop both feet back to plank.

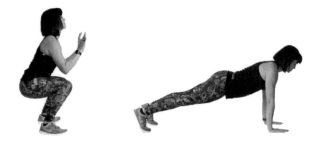

B Lower onto stomach, extend and lift arms and legs out to "Superman" position, then "swim" arms back and forth. Return to plank and finish with a vertical jump.

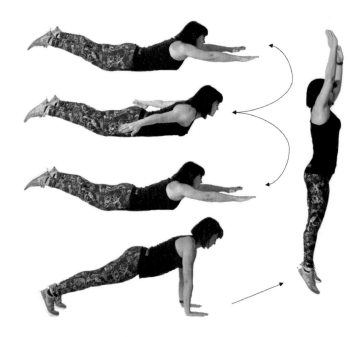

BURPEE VARIATION #54:

DEAD MAN BURPEE

A Squat, bring hands to floor and hop both feet back to plank.

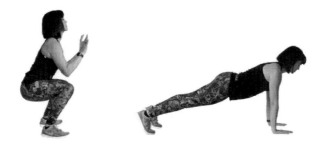

B Bend elbows and lower onto stomach. Extend both arms out to the sides. Bring them back to center and push-up to high plank. Hop feet to hands and jump straight up.

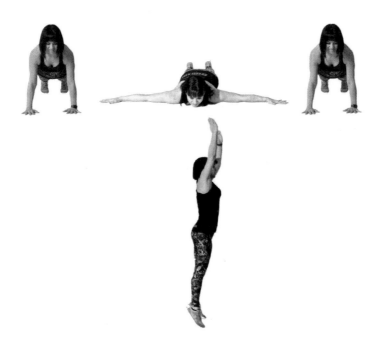

BURPEE VARIATION #55:

SQUAT JUMP SCISSOR BURPEE

A Squat, bring hands to floor, hop feet back to plank, push-up and jump.

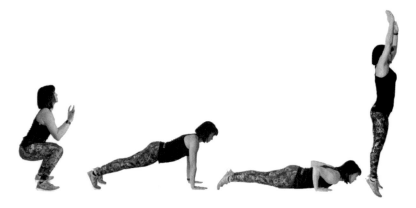

B Land from the jump into a squat, explode up and scissor legs, land in a squat and repeat the explosive scissor jump a second time and land in a squat. Feet together to end the burpee.

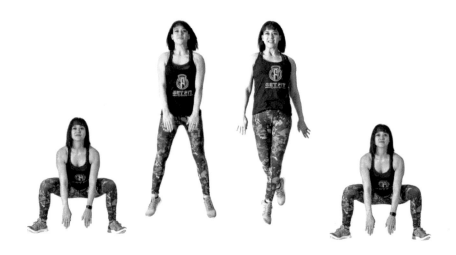

TRAINER'S TIP: Have client touch feet together instead of scissoring during the squat jump for a regression.

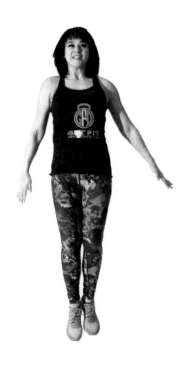

BURPEE VARIATION #56:

SINGLE LEG PUSH-UP BURPEE

A Squat, bring hands to floor and hop both feet back to plank.

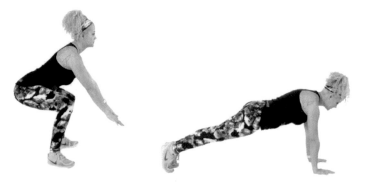

B From the plank, extend and lift one leg up. Complete a push-up with leg lifted. Return to plank, bring feet to hands and jump straight up. Repeat Steps A and B with the leg lift on the opposite side.

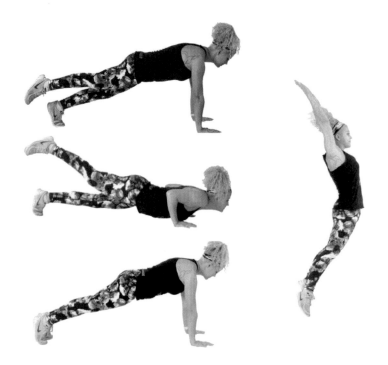

BURPEE VARIATION #57:

STAGGERED JUMP BURPEE

A Squat, bring hands to floor, hop feet back to plank, push-up.

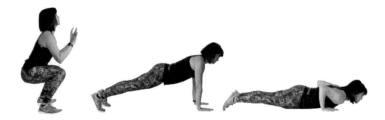

B Hop feet back towards hands in a staggered stance, one foot in front of the other. Proceed to jump and land with feet staggered.

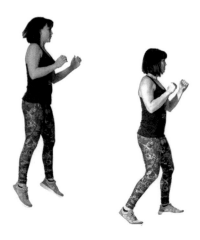

C Repeat Steps A and B, switching which leg is in front each staggered jump.

BURPEE VARIATION #58:

ROLLING BURPEE

A Squat, bring hands to floor and hop both feet back to plank.

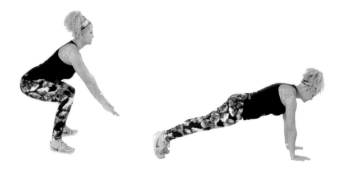

B Bend elbows and lower onto stomach. Extend both arms out in front of body, then roll to one side until you are back on your stomach.

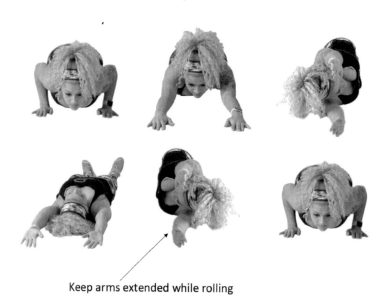

Keep arms extended while rolling

C Push up to plank, hop feet to hands and jump up. Repeat Steps A and B—rolling to the other side.

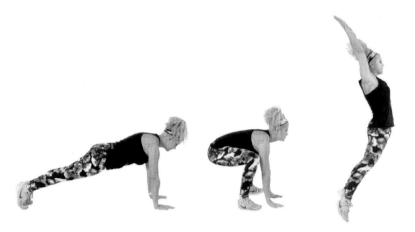

BURPEE VARIATION #59:

SINGLE LEG DEADLIFT HOP BURPEE

A Lift one knee up, balancing on the other leg. Slowly bring that knee down and extend leg behind you.

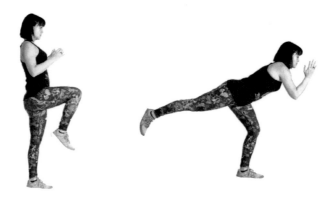

B Bend knee and bring it back up, using momentum to complete a single leg hop. Drop down and perform a single leg plank and push-up.

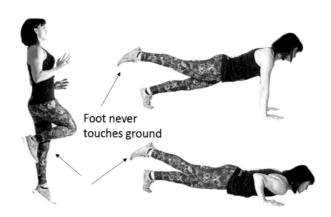

Foot never touches ground

C Bring lifted foot down, hop both feet back to hands, and jump straight up. Repeat the entire sequence on the other leg.

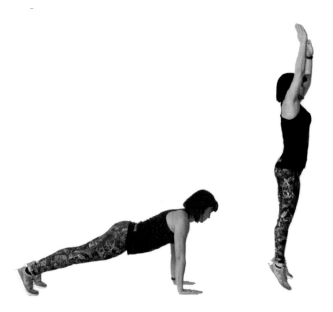

TRAINER'S TIP: Have client focus on balance and strength, not speed. Use other arm and swing up to aid in gaining momentum for the hop.

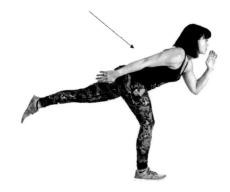

BURPEE VARIATION #60:

SIDE SPRAWL BURPEE

A Sprawl diagonally, hips and thighs towards floor and head up. Jump up, repeat sprawl to the other side.

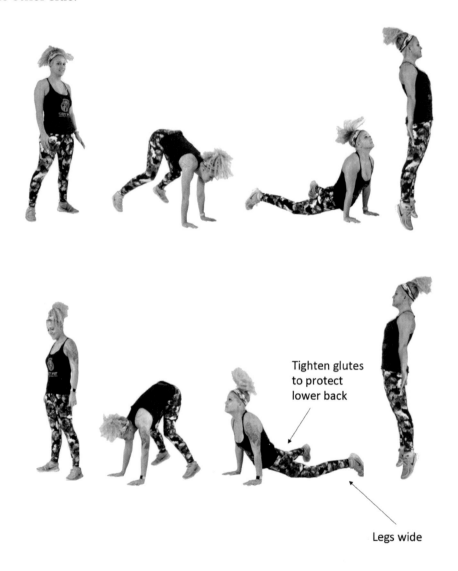

Tighten glutes to protect lower back

Legs wide

BURPEE VARIATION #61:

SPRINTER BURPEE

A Squat, bring hands to floor, hop feet back to plank and push-up .

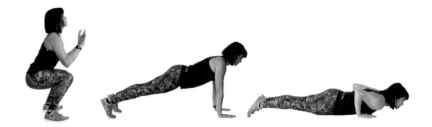

B Hop both feet back to hands, jump up and sprint as fast as you can for 4 reps.

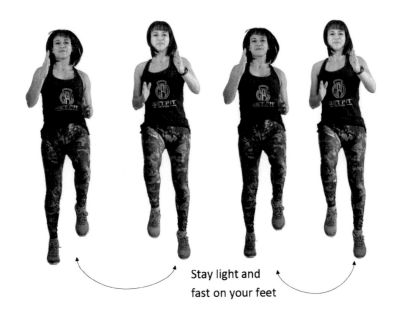

Stay light and
fast on your feet

BURPEE VARIATION #62:

A CIRCLE OF BURPEES

A Perform 4-5 burpees in a circle. As you come out of each jump, push off to the right side (counterclockwise). Reverse the motion and burpee in a circle to the left next rotation (clockwise).

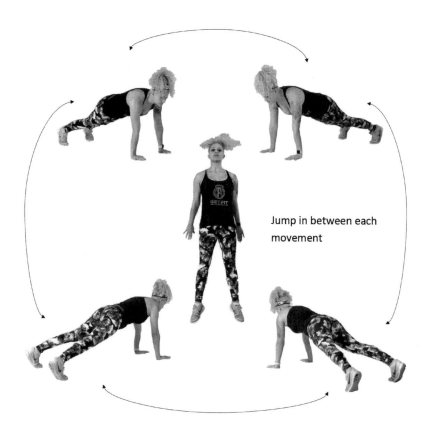

Jump in between each movement

TRAINER'S TIP: Add a push-up at the bottom of the movement each time you rotate to increase difficulty.

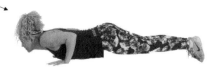

BURPEE VARIATION #63:

KNEE STRIKE BURPEE

A Send hips forward and bend knee while bringing your heel towards your bottom for a knee strike.

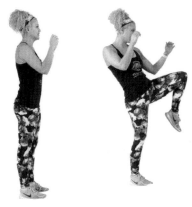

B Bring foot down after knee strike. Squat, bring hands to floor and hop feet back to plank and push-up.

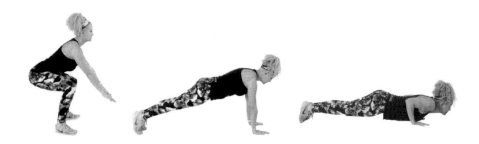

C Bring feet back to hands and jump straight up. Land and immediately execute a knee strike with the other leg. Repeat for as many reps as you want, switching knees in between each burpee.

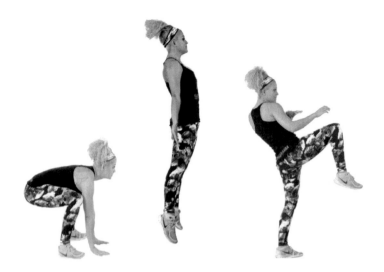

BURPEE VARIATION #64:

TRAVELLING PLYO PUSH-UP BURPEE

A Squat, bring hands to floor and hop feet back to plank.

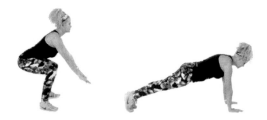

B Bend elbows and knees as you lower yourself to the floor in a hover. Push explosively off both hands and feet while moving forward in a "hopping" motion. Repeat 2-3 more times moving forward. Bring feet to hands and end the burpee with a jump.

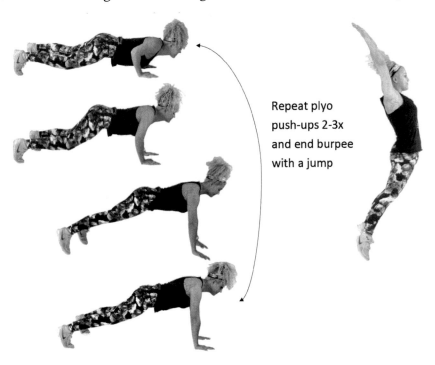

Repeat plyo push-ups 2-3x and end burpee with a jump

TRAINER'S TIP: This exercise is for advanced clients only.

BURPEE VARIATION #65:

LATERAL HOP & LUNGE BURPEE

A Hop to the right, step left leg back and lunge. Quickly bring leg back and hop to the left side and repeat lunge with right leg.

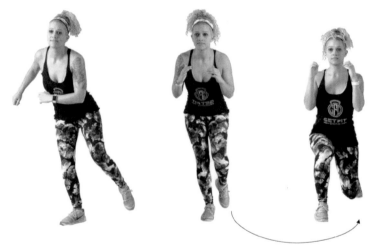

Inside leg touches floor lightly then lunges back

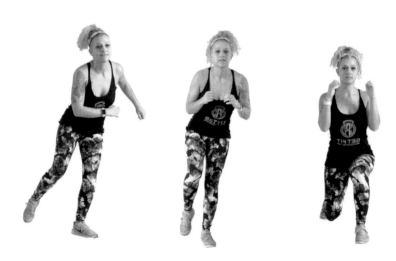

A Bring both feet together, then do a regular burpee all the way through including the jump.

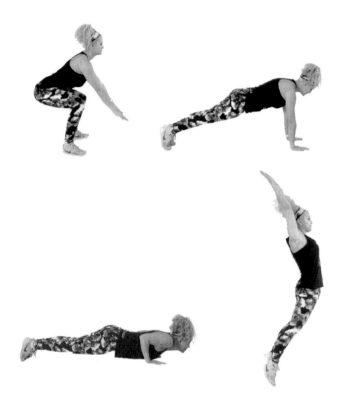

TRAINER'S TIP: Make it harder by adding jumping lunges after each lateral hop.

BURPEE VARIATION #66:

WIDE LEGGED BURPEE

A Bend knees and bring hands to floor, hop both feet back to a wide legged "V"

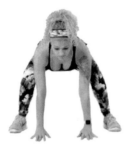 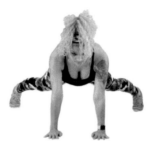

TRAINER'S TIP: Add a push-up while feet are wide for difficulty

B Keeping legs wide, hop both feet back to hands and finish with a vertical jump.

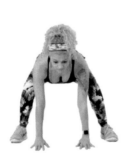 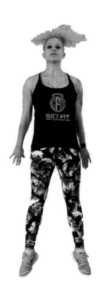

BURPEE VARIATION #67:

ALTERNATING LEG RAISE BURPEE

A Squat, bring hands to floor and hop both feet back to plank.

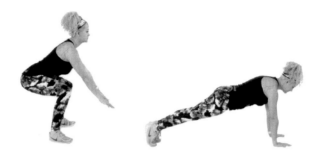

B Bend elbows and start a push-up. As you lower yourself, bring one leg up and complete the push-up. Set leg down and repeat push-up while raising the other leg. Set foot down

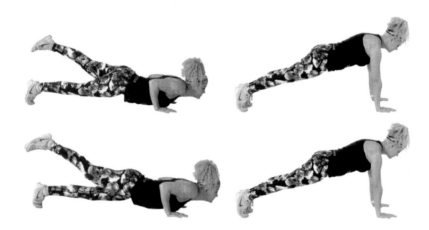

BURPEE VARIATION #68:

YIPPEE KAI YAY BURPEE

A Squat, bring hands to floor and hop both feet back to plank.

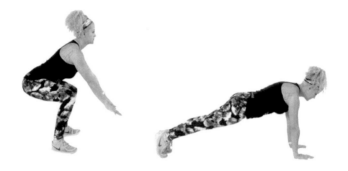

B From the plank, kick one leg out to the side and let the other leg follow in a hopping motion. Hop one leg at a time back to the middle and then repeat kick and hop to the other side.

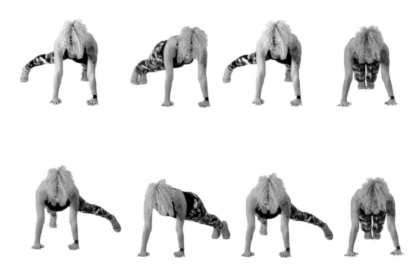

C Hop both feet back to hands and jump up to finish the burpee.

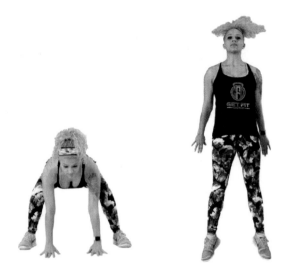

BURPEE VARIATION #69:

DROP IT LIKE A SQUAT BURPEE

A You will start and end this burpee in a squat. From the squat, step back with the right leg in a lunging motion, then bring leg back to squat. Repeat with the left leg and bring back to squat. Stay low.

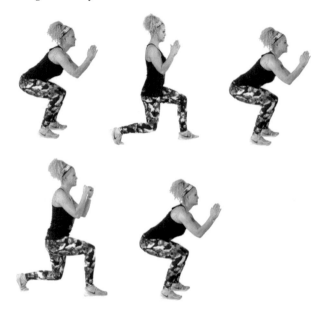

B From the squat, bring hands to floor and hop both feet back to plank and then back to hands. End in a squat.

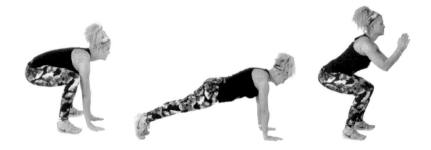

C Hop both feet back to hands and jump up to finish the burpee.

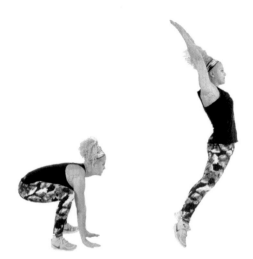

PART 2
BURPEE VARIATIONS CONTINUED

BURPEES USING VARIOUS TYPES OF EQUIPMENT

IN THIS SECTION, we show a few variations you can try using equipment most personal trainers have access to. Use common sense and caution, as it may not be safe to do some of these with clients who are just starting a fitness routine and those who don't have the strength yet.

There are so many we couldn't fit in this book, so feel free to let these inspire you to create your own variations.

BURPEE VARIATION #70:

WEIGHTED VEST BURPEE

Equipment needed: Weighted vest of choice

A Choose a weighted vest according to client fitness level. We like 20 lbs. or more. Perform a full burpee with the added resistance.

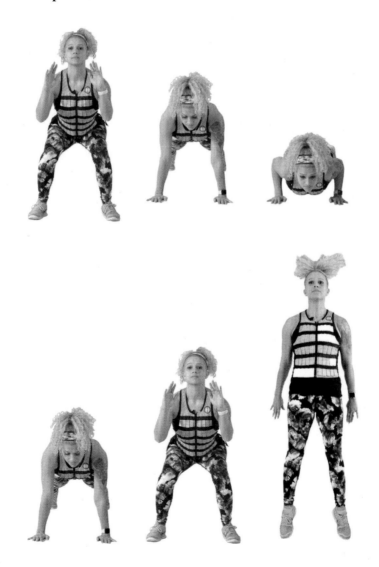

BURPEE VARIATION #71:

KNEES TO ELBOW BURPEE

Equipment needed: Sturdy pull-up bar rig. Plyo box for regression or assistance.

A Start by facing a pull-up bar. Drop down, do a burpee with a push-up. Drive up and catch the pull-up bar on the jump. Bring knees to elbows and down. Slowly release bar and land softly.

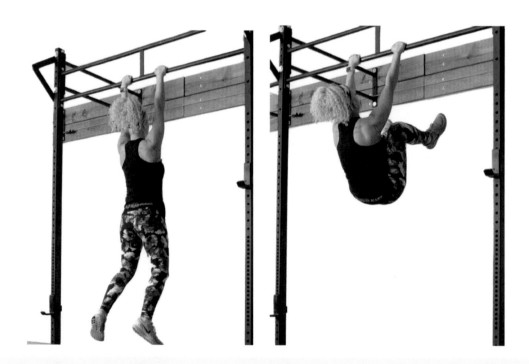

TRAINER'S TIP: Overhand or underhand grip is fine depending on goals and client.

B Variation/regression: Use a plyo box for clients less advanced or for assistance to get to and from the pull-up bar. Jump or step onto the box to get to the pull-up bar.

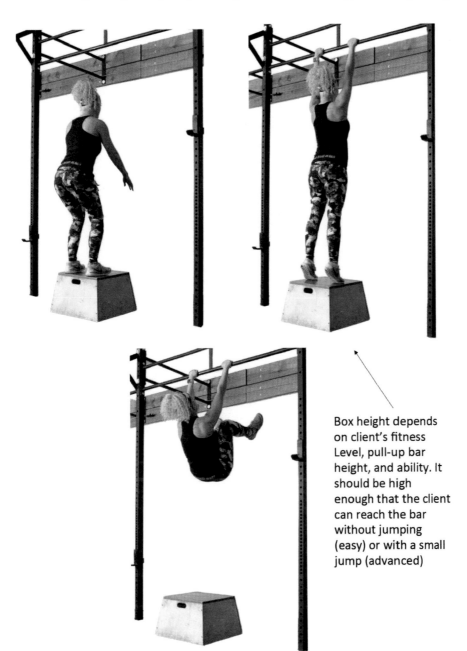

Box height depends on client's fitness Level, pull-up bar height, and ability. It should be high enough that the client can reach the bar without jumping (easy) or with a small jump (advanced)

BURPEE VARIATION #72:

PULL-UP BURPEE

Equipment needed: Sturdy pull-up bar rig. Plyo box for regression or assistance.

 Start by facing a pull-up bar. Drop down, do a burpee with a push-up. Drive up and catch the pull-up bar on the jump. Do one pull-up. Lower slowly and release bar.

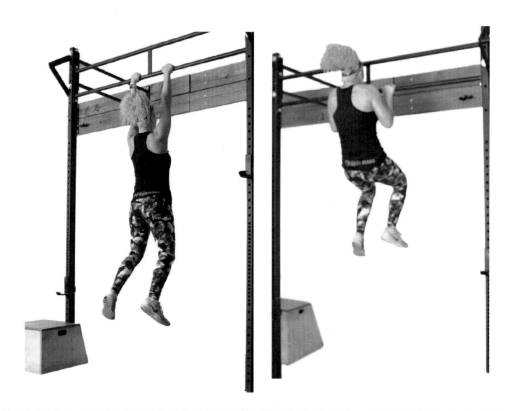

TRAINER'S TIP: Overhand or underhand grip is fine depending on goals and client.

B **Variation/regression:** Use a plyo box for clients less advanced or for assistance to get to and from the pull-up bar. Jump or step onto the box to get to the pull-up bar.

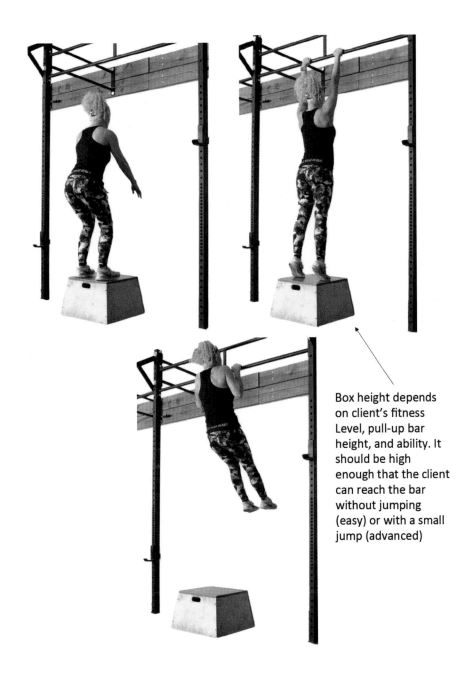

Box height depends on client's fitness Level, pull-up bar height, and ability. It should be high enough that the client can reach the bar without jumping (easy) or with a small jump (advanced)

BURPEE VARIATION #73:

LADDER BURPEE

Equipment needed: Fitness ladder

A In and out footwork (shuffle and alternate feet) down the fitness ladder. Do a regular burpee at the end. Repeat in and out footwork back to start, regular burpee. For longer ladders, you can do a burpee every 3 rungs or so.

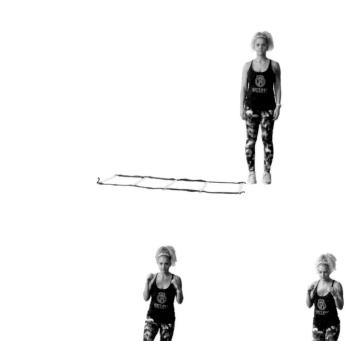

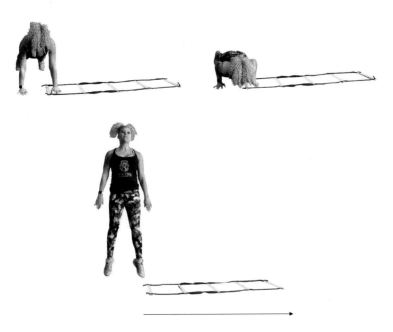

Repeat sequence back and end with a regular burpee

TRAINER'S TIP: There are lots of way to add variety. Change up the footwork sequence, the amount of burpees, etc.

BURPEE VARIATION #74:

INCLINE BOX BURPEE

Equipment needed: 12-24" Sturdy plyo box . Sub any sturdy elevated surface.

A Start facing a sturdy box or other elevated surface. Place hands on the top of the box, hop or walk both feet back to a plank and do an incline push-up. Hop both feet back towards hands and jump up in front of the box.

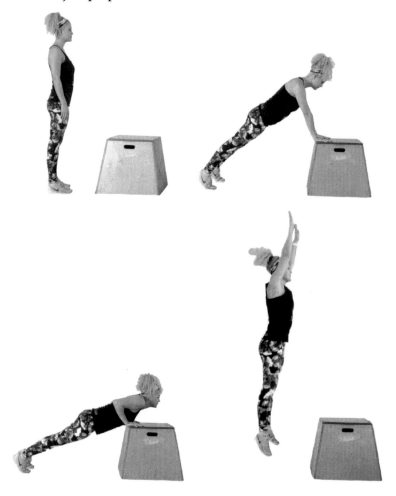

TRAINER'S TIP: This is a great modification for clients who need a little help with push-ups or are starting out. Eliminate the push-up and/or the jump for further regression.

BURPEE VARIATION #75:

BOX JUMP BURPEE

Equipment needed: 12"-24" Sturdy plyo box (based on client level of ability)

A Start facing a sturdy plyo box. Make sure you have some space in front of the box. Drop down and do a regular burpee through the push-up. Bring feet to hands and continue to drive up and forward to land with both feet on top of the box.

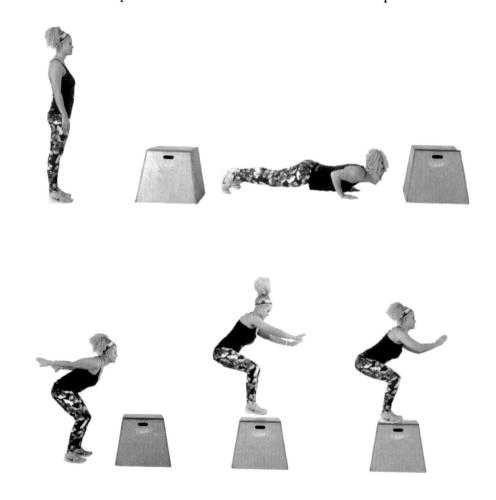

B Make sure both feet are planted and you can stand completely stable before bending knees and jumping back down to end the burpee.

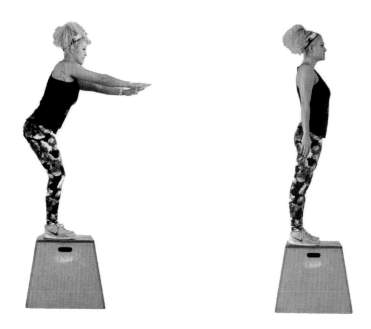

TRAINER'S TIP: Introduce or modify this burpee with a step up onto the box instead of a jump and/or a step down (easier to learn where your center of gravity is and foot placement)

BURPEE VARIATION #76:

LATERAL BOX STEP BURPEE

Equipment needed: 12" Sturdy plyo box (max height recommended)

A Start to the side of the box. Shuffle or step up one foot at a time and move laterally to the other side of the box. Drop down and push-up. Repeat lateral box sequence to return to starting side, drop down and push-up to finish the burpee.

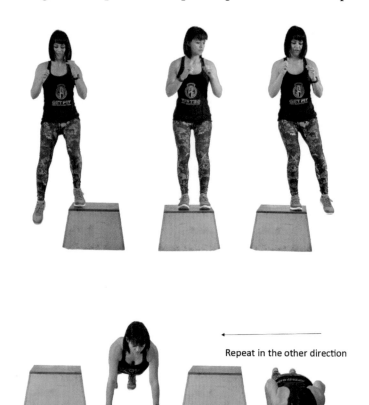

Repeat in the other direction

TRAINER'S TIP: Shuffling or a quicker movement is for more advanced students. Be cautious with foot placement and make sure both feet touch the box in transition.

BURPEE VARIATION #77:

TOE TAP BURPEE

Equipment needed: 12" Sturdy plyo box (max height recommended)

A Stand directly in front of a low box. Quickly alternate toe tapping feet on the top of the box 4-5 times.

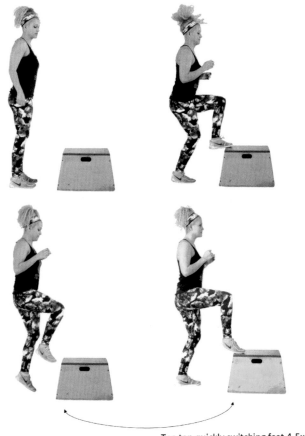

Toe tap quickly switching feet 4-5x

B Place hands on box, do an incline push-up and then jump up in front of the box to finish the burpee.

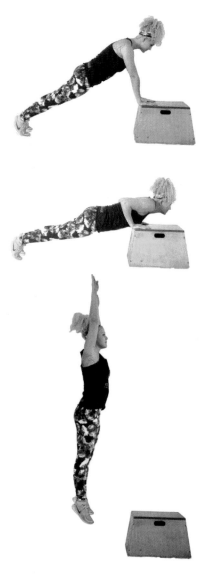

BURPEE VARIATION #78:

KNEE UP BOX BURPEE

Equipment needed: 12-24" Sturdy plyo box (depends on client height and flexibility)

A Start by standing directly in front of a plyo box. Step on the box with one foot, push off heel and lift other leg up while bringing knee up. Step down with the leg you lifted the knee up with. Repeat with the other leg.

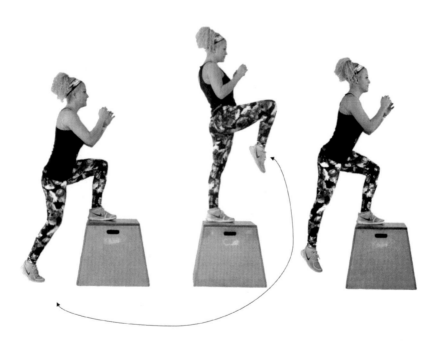

Keep that foot off the floor and use the opposite leg to go up and down the box

B Place hands on the box in front of you and do an incline push-up. Jump up in front of the box to finish the burpee.

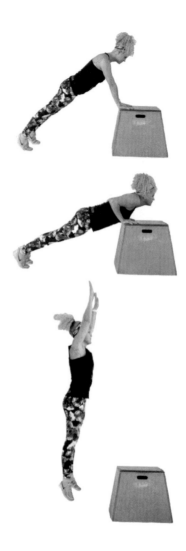

BURPEE VARIATION #79:

DECLINE BOX BURPEE

Equipment needed: 12-24" Sturdy plyo box (vary height according to client fitness level)

A Start by standing facing away from a plyo box (back towards box). Bring hands towards floor and hop both feet back and up onto the plyo box into a decline plank.

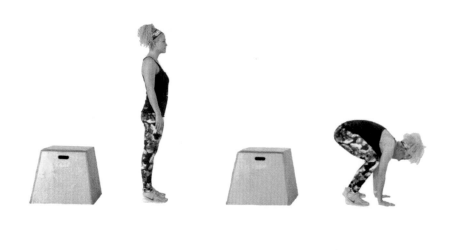

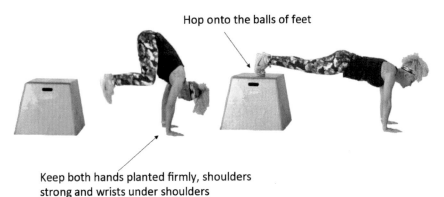

Hop onto the balls of feet

Keep both hands planted firmly, shoulders strong and wrists under shoulders

B From the decline plank, do a push-up. Return to plank and hop both feet off the box and back to hands. Finish the burpee with a vertical jump.

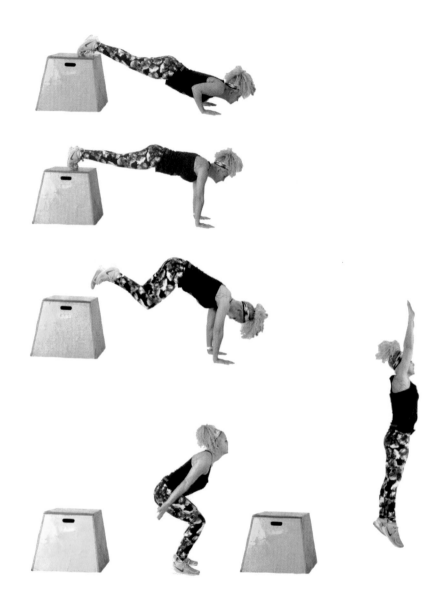

TRAINER'S TIP: Difficult burpee-Modify by stepping one foot up at a time onto the box.

BURPEE VARIATION #80:

BOX OF DEATH BURPEE

Equipment needed: 12-24" Sturdy plyo box (vary height according to client fitness level)

A Start by standing directly in front of a plyo box. Jump onto the box, making sure both feet are planted, then jump laterally off the box to the right. Perform a push-up.

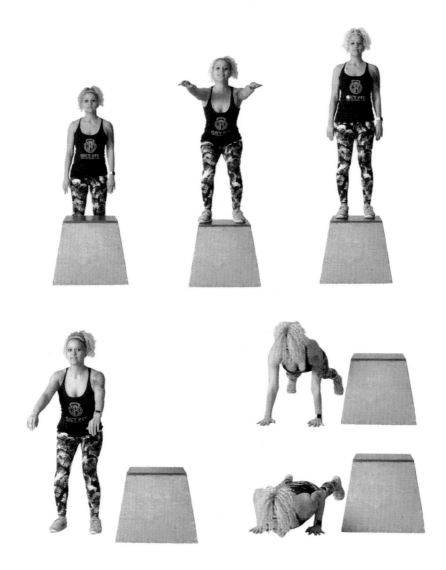

B Jump laterally back onto the box, making sure feet are planted. Jump backwards off the box (where you started) then immediately back on. Jump laterally off the box to the left. Push-up.

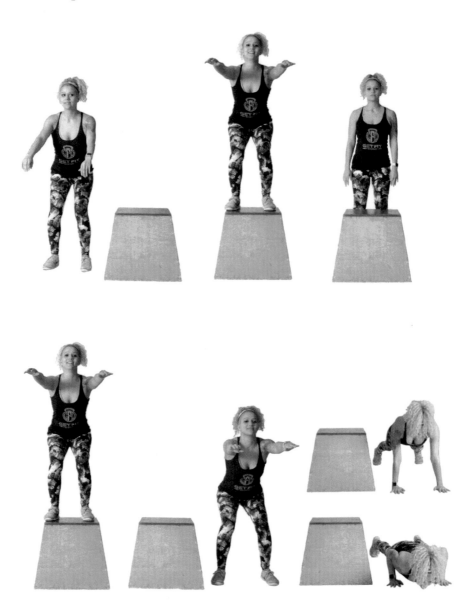

C Jump laterally back onto the box, Jump backwards off the box to end the burpee where you began.

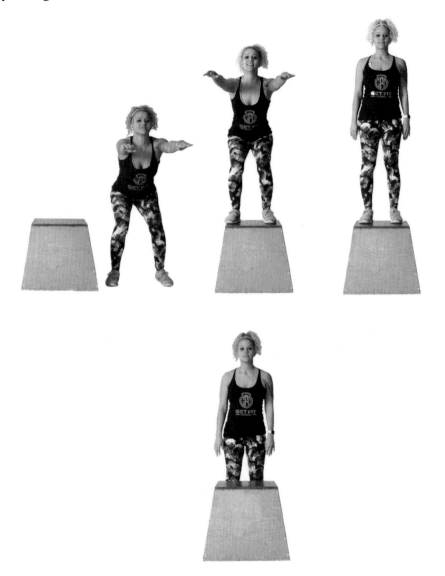

TRAINER'S TIP: Not recommended for clients with knee or balance issues. All jumps can be modified by stepping on and off the box for a good regression. Start with a low box.

BURPEE VARIATION #81:

BATTLE ROPE WAVE BURPEE

Equipment needed: 30-40' Battle Rope

A From a 1/2 squat position, hold the battle rope in both hands. Do 4-5 up and down "waves" with the rope.

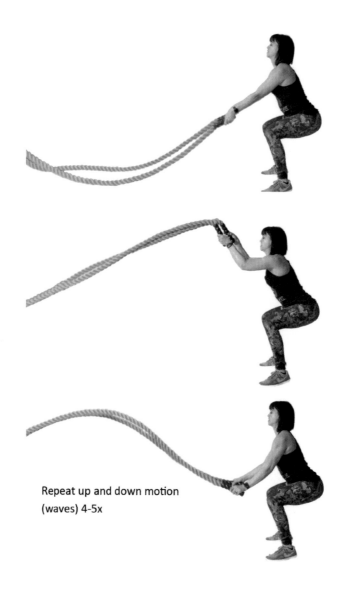

Repeat up and down motion (waves) 4-5x

B Drop down to plank, push-up, then hop back up and jump (hold onto the rope).

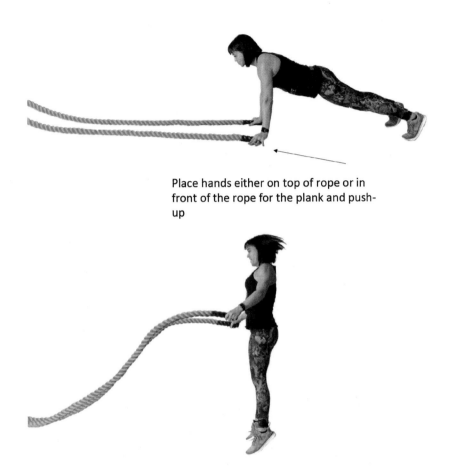

Place hands either on top of rope or in front of the rope for the plank and push-up

TRAINER'S TIP: Beginners can just practice the rope waves. Modify this burpee by adding or eliminating the push-up and the jump.

BURPEE VARIATION #82:

SINGLE ARM BATTLE ROPE WAVE BURPEE

Equipment needed: 30-40' Battle Rope

A From a 1/2 squat position, hold the battle rope in one hand. Do 4-5 up and down "waves" with the rope.

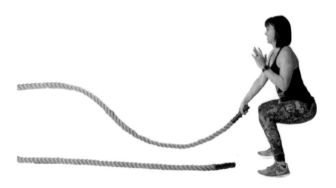

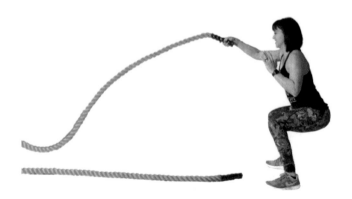

Repeat up and down motion
(waves) 4-5x

B Drop down to plank, push-up, then hop back up and jump (hold onto the rope with same single arm). Repeat Steps A-B with the other arm.

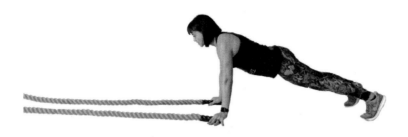

Place hands either on top of rope or in front of the rope for the plank and push-up

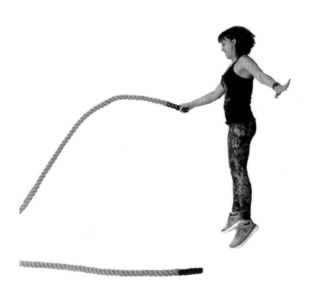

TRAINER'S TIP: Beginners can just practice the rope waves. Modify this burpee by adding or eliminating the push-up and the jump.

BURPEE VARIATION #83:

BATTLE ROPE DRUMMER BURPEE

Equipment needed: 30-40' Battle Rope

A From a 1/2 squat position, hold the battle rope in both hands. Do 4-6 "drummer" (alternating arms) waves with the rope.

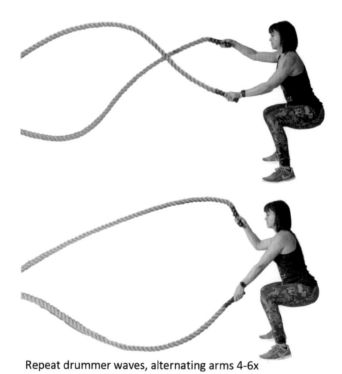

Repeat drummer waves, alternating arms 4-6x

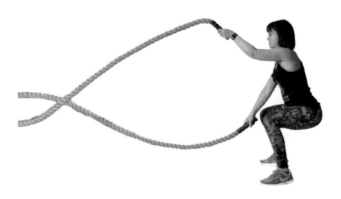

B Drop down to plank, push-up, then hop back up and jump (hold onto the rope).

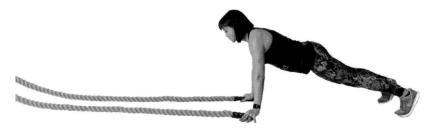

Place hands either on top of rope or in front of the rope for the plank and push-up

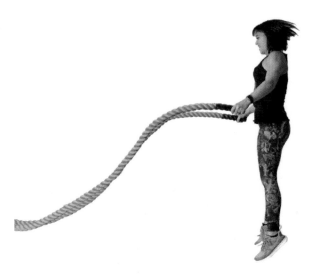

TRAINER'S TIP: Beginners can just practice the drumming. Modify this burpee by adding or eliminating the push-up and the jump.

BURPEE VARIATION #84:

DUMMY BAG DEADLIFT BURPEE

Equipment needed: 30-75 lb. dummy bag with handles, or sandbag with handles . Vary weight according to client fitness ability.

A Start by placing the dummy bag horizontally in front of you. Bend knees and place hands flat on the bag as you hop both legs back to plank. Perform a push-up.

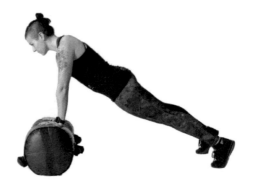

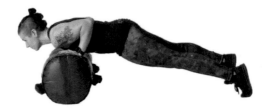

B Hop both feet back towards bag. Reach hands over and grab both outside handles. Let your arms hang like ropes. Don't pull with arms. Use your legs and hips and deadlift the bag. Finish with a small vertical jump.

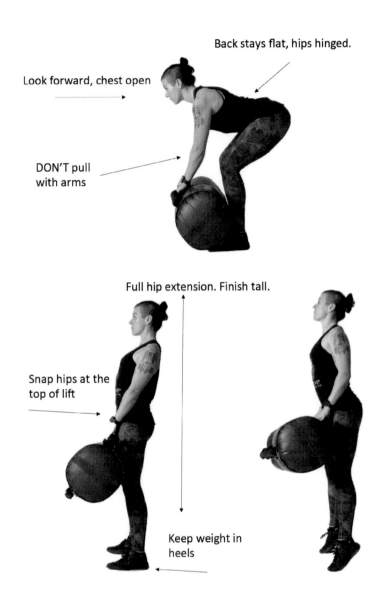

Back stays flat, hips hinged.

Look forward, chest open

DON'T pull with arms

Full hip extension. Finish tall.

Snap hips at the top of lift

Keep weight in heels

BURPEE VARIATION #85:

DUMMY BAG CLEAN & SQUAT BURPEE

Equipment needed: 30-75 lb. dummy bag with handles, or sandbag with handles . Vary weight according to client fitness ability.

 Follow the steps to deadlift the bag: Reach hands over and grab both outside handles. Let your arms hang like ropes. Don't pull with arms.

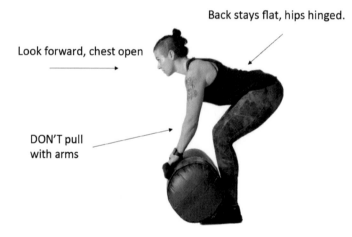

Back stays flat, hips hinged.

Look forward, chest open

DON'T pull with arms

B Clean: Aggressively drive both feet into the floor and snap hips as you shrug and high pull the bag, catching it on your forearms and biceps in a cradling motion.

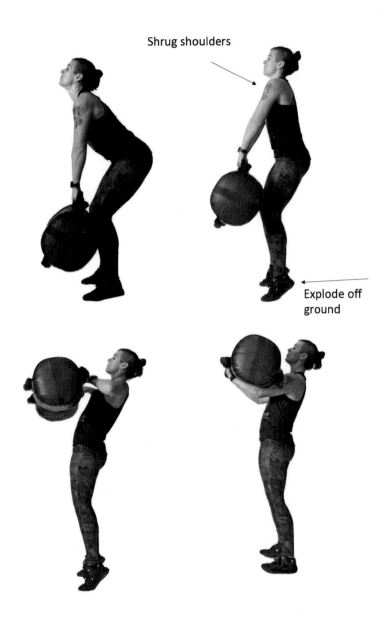

Shrug shoulders

Explode off
ground

C With the bag cradled in the nook of your forearms and biceps, squat down and back up.

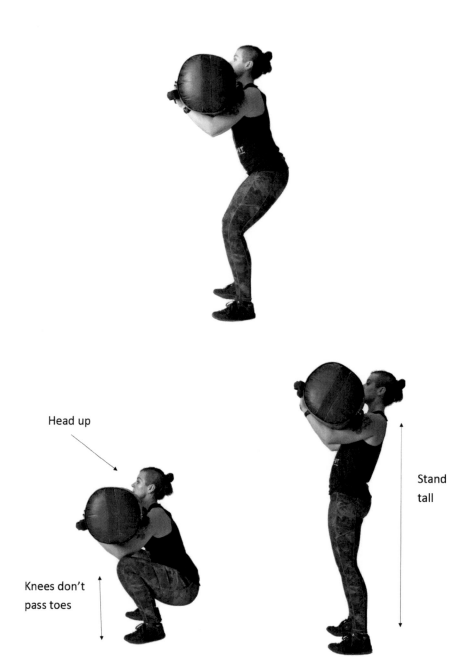

Head up

Knees don't pass toes

Stand tall

D Let bag unwind carefully down arms and lower bag to the floor in a reverse deadlift motion. Place hands on bag and perform a push-up.

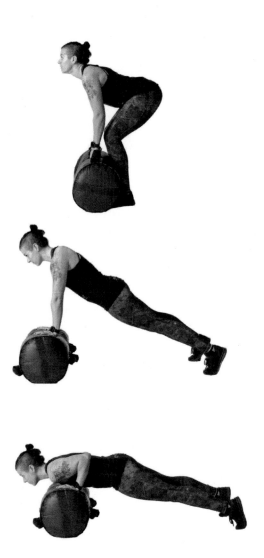

E Hop both feet back towards bag. Reach hands over and grab both outside handles. Let your arms hang like ropes. Don't pull with arms. Use your legs and hips and deadlift the bag. Finish with a small vertical jump.

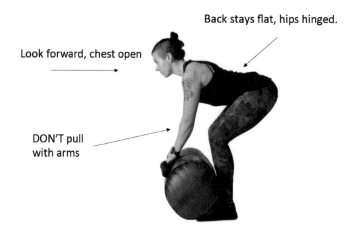

Back stays flat, hips hinged.

Look forward, chest open

DON'T pull with arms

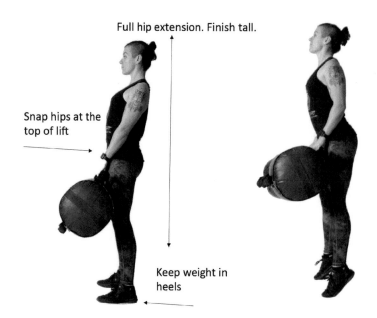

Full hip extension. Finish tall.

Snap hips at the top of lift

Keep weight in heels

BURPEE VARIATION #86:

DUMMY BAG CLEAN & PRESS BURPEE

Equipment needed: 30-75 lb. dummy bag with handles, or sandbag with handles . Vary weight according to client fitness ability.

 Follow the steps to deadlift the bag: Reach hands over and grab both outside handles. Let your arms hang like ropes. Don't pull with arms.

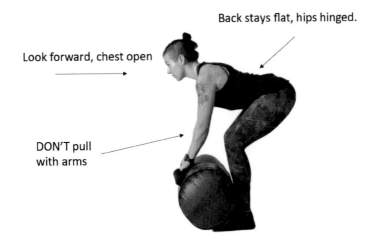

Look forward, chest open

Back stays flat, hips hinged.

DON'T pull with arms

B Clean: Aggressively drive both feet into the floor and snap hips as you shrug and high pull the bag, catching it on your forearms and biceps.

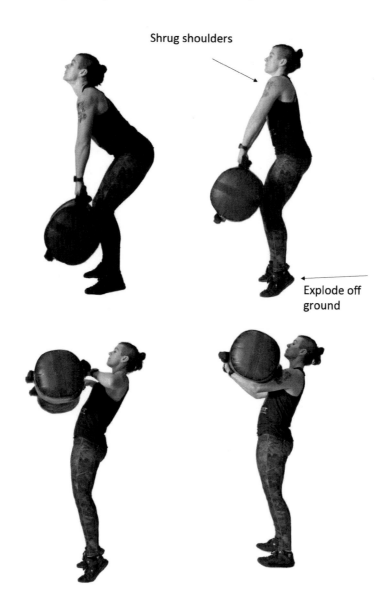

Shrug shoulders

Explode off ground

C Keep core tight and press bag overhead. Biceps stay close to ears and shoulders packed. Bag will be behind head.

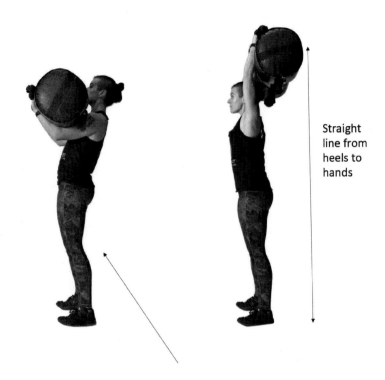

Straight line from heels to hands

TRAINER'S TIP: Client can "dip" before pressing to assist and get the bag overhead. This is a dip, drive through heels and arms and press motion. Beginners can practice up to the clean and eliminate the press. If needed, release bag so that it falls behind you.

D Bring the bag back to the cradle position, then let the bag unwind down arms as you lower bag to the floor in a reverse deadlift. Place hands on bag and perform a push-up.

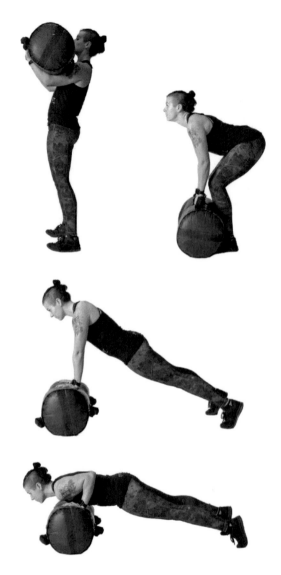

E Hop both feet back towards bag. Reach hands over and grab both outside handles. Let your arms hang like ropes. Don't pull with arms. Use your legs and hips and deadlift the bag. Finish with a small vertical jump.

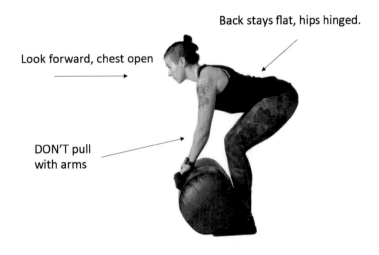

Look forward, chest open

Back stays flat, hips hinged.

DON'T pull with arms

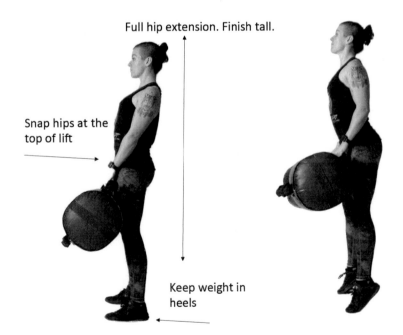

Full hip extension. Finish tall.

Snap hips at the top of lift

Keep weight in heels

BURPEE VARIATION #87:

DUMMY BAG CLEAN, SQUAT & PRESS BURPEE

Equipment needed: 30-75 lb. dummy bag with handles, or sandbag with handles . Vary weight according to client fitness ability.

 Follow the steps to deadlift the bag: Reach hands over and grab both outside handles. Let your arms hang like ropes. Don't pull with arms.

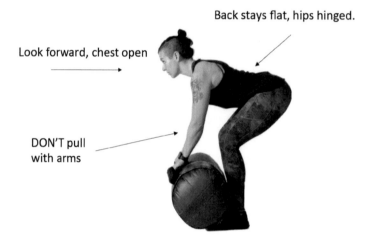

Look forward, chest open

Back stays flat, hips hinged.

DON'T pull with arms

B Clean: Aggressively drive both feet into the floor and snap hips as you shrug and high pull the bag, catching it on your forearms and biceps.

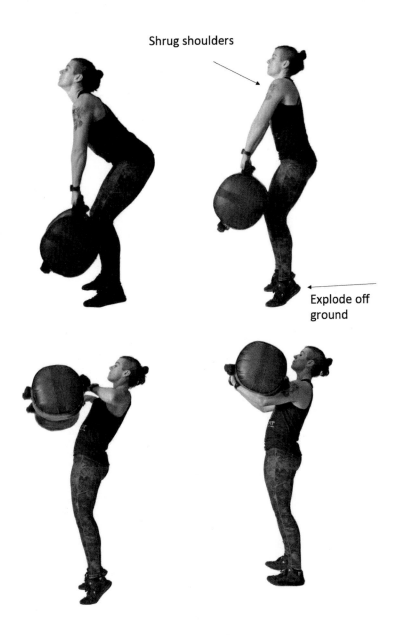

Shrug shoulders

Explode off ground

C With the bag cradled in the nook of your forearms and biceps, squat down and back up.

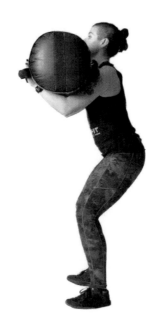

Head up

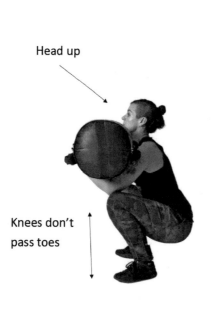

Knees don't pass toes

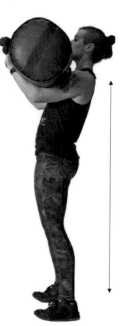

Stand tall

D Keep core tight and press bag overhead. Biceps stay close to ears and shoulders packed. Bag will be behind head.

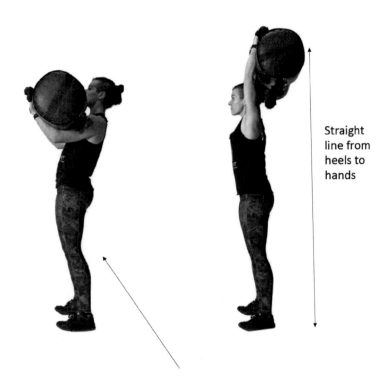

Straight line from heels to hands

TRAINER'S TIP: Client can "dip" before pressing to assist and get the bag overhead. This is a dip , drive through heels and arms and press motion. Beginners can practice up to the clean and eliminate the press. If needed, release bag so that it falls behind you.

E Bring the bag back to the cradle position, then let the bag unwind down arms as you lower bag to the floor in a reverse deadlift . Place hands on bag and perform a push-up.

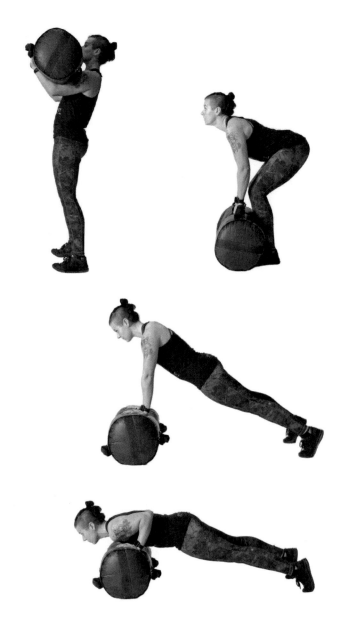

F Hop both feet back towards bag. Reach hands over and grab both outside handles. Let your arms hang like ropes. Don't pull with arms. Use your legs and hips and deadlift the bag. Finish with a small vertical jump.

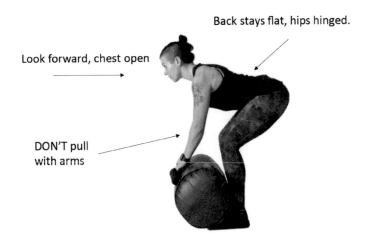

Look forward, chest open

Back stays flat, hips hinged.

DON'T pull with arms

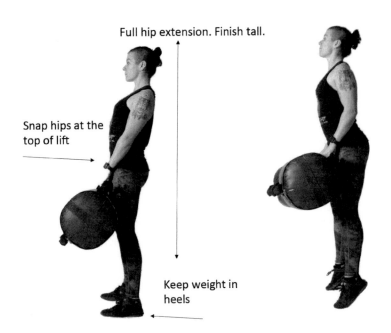

Full hip extension. Finish tall.

Snap hips at the top of lift

Keep weight in heels

BURPEE VARIATION #88:

DUMMY BAG ROW BURPEE

Equipment needed: 30-75 lb. dummy bag with handles, or sandbag with handles . Vary weight according to client fitness ability.

A Start by placing the dummy bag horizontally in front of you. Rotate handles up towards you. Bend knees, back flat, and grab both handles. Squeeze shoulder blades and bring elbows back as you row the bag towards midsection. Repeat rowing motion twice.

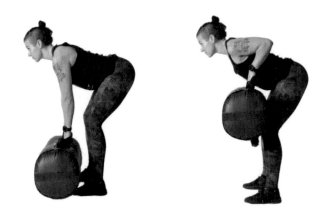

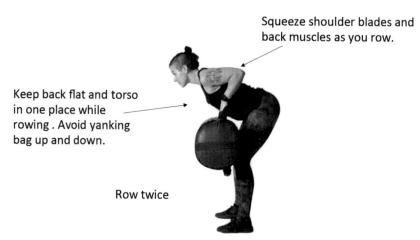

Squeeze shoulder blades and back muscles as you row.

Keep back flat and torso in one place while rowing . Avoid yanking bag up and down.

Row twice

B Place bag on the floor and let go of the handles. Place hands on bag and perform a push-up.

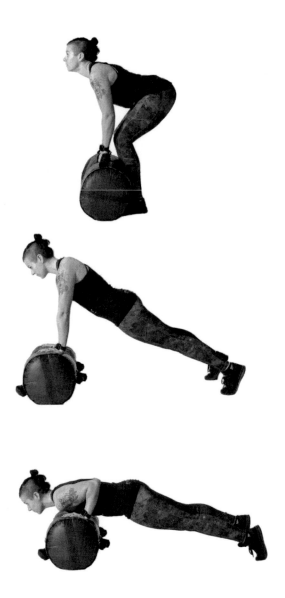

C Hop both feet back towards bag. Reach hands over and grab both outside handles. Let your arms hang like ropes. Don't pull with arms. Use your legs and hips and deadlift the bag. Finish with a small vertical jump.

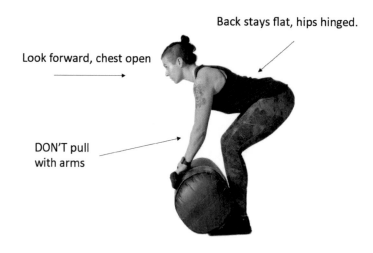

Back stays flat, hips hinged.

Look forward, chest open

DON'T pull with arms

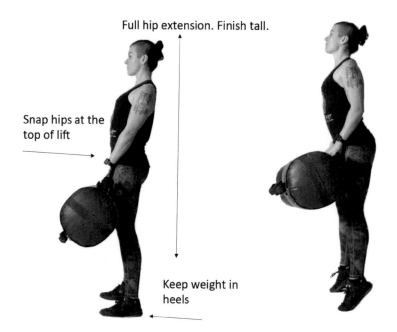

Full hip extension. Finish tall.

Snap hips at the top of lift

Keep weight in heels

BURPEE VARIATION #89:

DUMMY BAG FIREMAN CARRY BURPEE

Equipment needed: 30-75 lb. dummy bag with handles, or sandbag with handles . Vary weight according to client fitness ability.

A Start by placing the dummy bag perpendicular to you. Straddle the bag, sit on it, grab both sides.

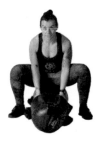

B Lift the bag up and over one shoulder as you stand. Keep the bag close to your body as you swing it up and over.

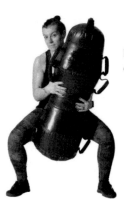

Keep bag close to you

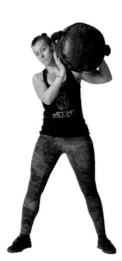

C Swing the bag back down the floor. Place hands on the bag and kick feet behind you. Do a push-up on the bag.

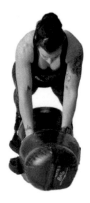
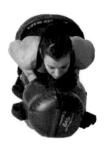

D Hop feet to straddle the bag. Jump up into a knee tuck and land straddled. Repeat fireman lift burpee on the other side.

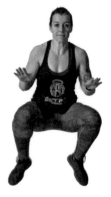
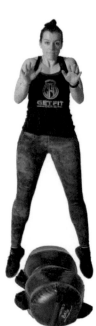

TRAINER'S TIP: Advanced burpee. Add a squat after the lift to make it more difficult. Add walking a few steps after the lift for added difficulty.

BURPEE VARIATION #90:

MEDICINE BALL BURPEE

Equipment needed: 10-20 lb. medicine ball or weight according to client fitness ability.

A Start by holding a medicine ball of choice at chest or hip height. Squat and lower medicine ball to the floor. Keeping hands on ball, hop both feet back to plank do a stability push-up.

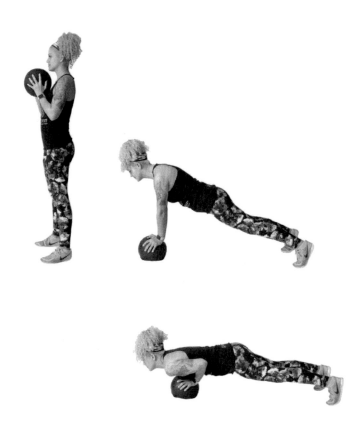

B Hop both feet back towards hands and deadlift the ball up. Continue the motion and jump straight up, holding the medicine ball at hip height during the jump.

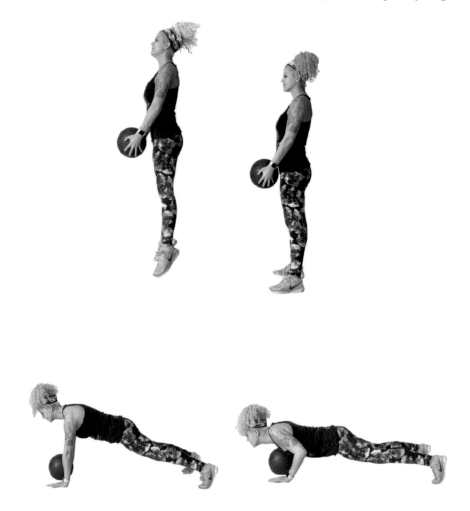

TRAINER'S TIP: This requires core strength. If client cannot do a push-up with hands on the ball, simply have them release the ball and then place hands on either side instead of on the ball.

BURPEE VARIATION #91:

MEDICINE BALL STAGGERED PUSH-UP BURPEE

Equipment needed: 10-20 lb. medicine ball or weight according to client fitness ability.

 Start by holding a medicine ball of choice at chest or hip height. Squat and lower medicine ball to the floor. Keeping hands on ball, hop both feet back to plank.

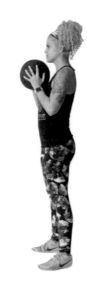

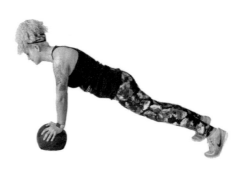

B Stagger hands so that one is one the ball and one is off. Do a push-up. Hop both feet towards hands, grab ball with both hands and jump up, ball at hip height. Repeat Steps A-B on the other arm.

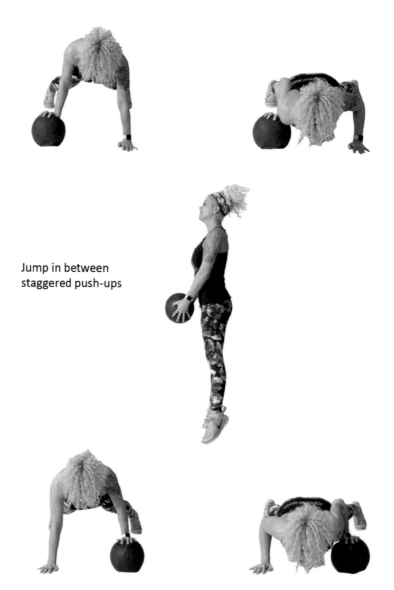

Jump in between staggered push-ups

BURPEE VARIATION #92:

MEDICINE BALL SLAM BURPEE

Equipment needed: 10-20 lb. medicine ball or weight according to client fitness ability.

A Start by holding a medicine ball at chest height and press to overhead position. Slam ball down to the floor, hinging from hips as you slam.

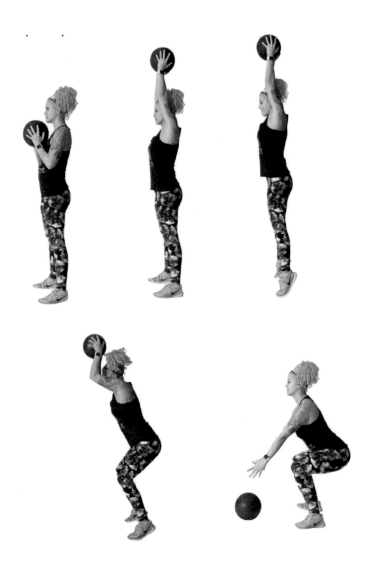

B Bring hands to floor on either side of the ball, push-up. Hop feet to hands, grab ball and jump straight up. Keep the ball at hip level on the jump.

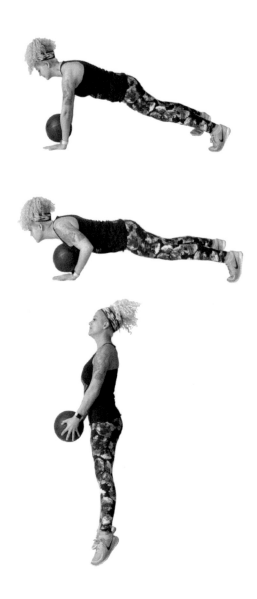

BURPEE VARIATION #93:

MEDICINE BALL SLURPEE BURPEE

Equipment needed: 10-20 lb. medicine ball or weight according to client fitness ability.

A Start by holding a medicine ball at chest height. Bend knees, squat and sit down and back. Continue momentum into a reverse crunch.

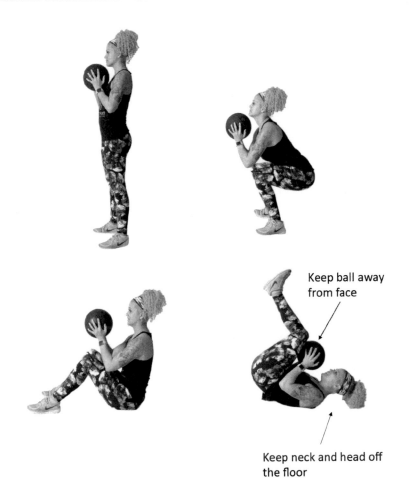

Keep ball away from face

Keep neck and head off the floor

B Rock forward from reverse crunch, keep feet close to bottom and come up to a low squat. Immediately flip into a stability ball plank. Do a push-up.

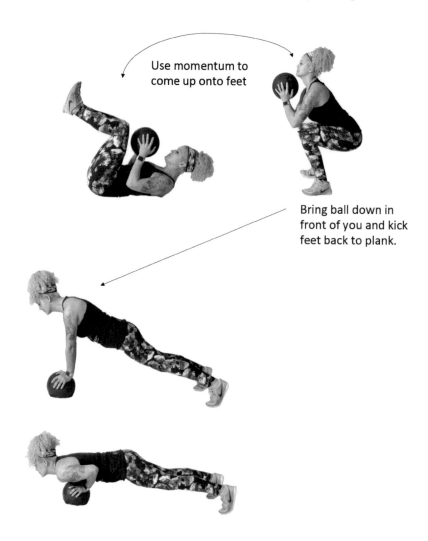

Use momentum to come up onto feet

Bring ball down in front of you and kick feet back to plank.

C Hop both feet back to hands, press ball up as you jump to end the burpee.

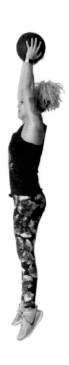

BURPEE VARIATION #94:

MEDICINE BALL SLURPEE BURPEE WALL BALL

Equipment needed: 10-20 lb. medicine ball or weight according to client fitness ability.

 Start by holding a medicine ball at chest height. Bend knees, squat and sit down and back. Continue momentum into a reverse crunch.

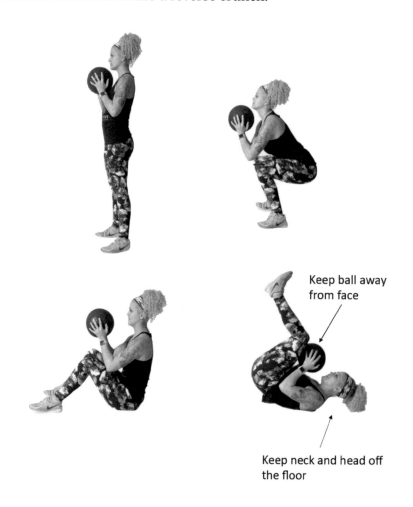

Keep ball away from face

Keep neck and head off the floor

B Rock forward from reverse crunch, keep feet close to bottom and come up to a low squat. Toss ball up to marked height, catch ball and squat down and back up to end the burpee.

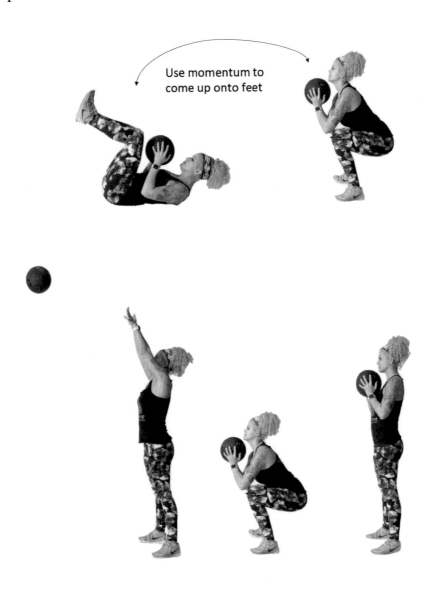

Use momentum to come up onto feet

BURPEE VARIATION #95:

MEDICINE BALL SLURPEE BURPEE BALL SLAM

Equipment needed: 10-20 lb. medicine ball or weight according to client fitness ability.

 Start by holding a medicine ball at chest height. Bend knees, squat and sit down and back. Continue momentum into a reverse crunch.

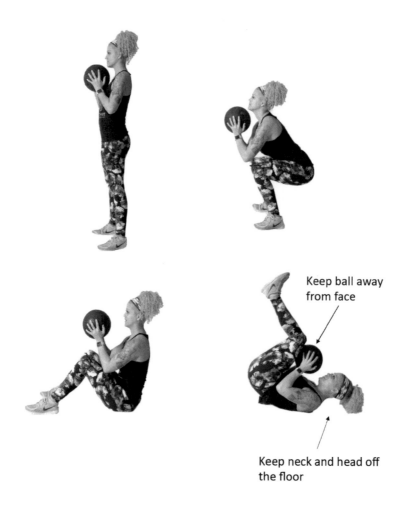

Keep ball away from face

Keep neck and head off the floor

B Rock forward from reverse crunch, keep feet close to bottom and go from squat to standing. Press ball overhead, then slam ball down to end the burpee.

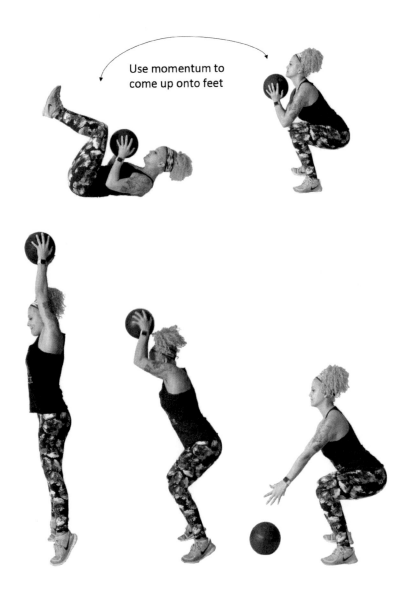

Use momentum to come up onto feet

BURPEE VARIATION #96:

AB WHEEL ROLLOUT BURPEE

Equipment needed: Sturdy Ab Wheel

A Start by holding an ab wheel low. Bend knees and place ab wheel on the floor in front of you.

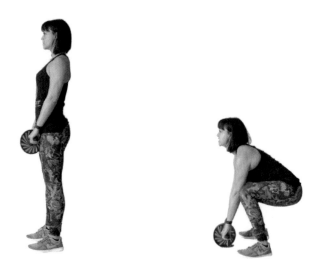

B Roll SLOWLY onto knees first, then out forward as far as you can.

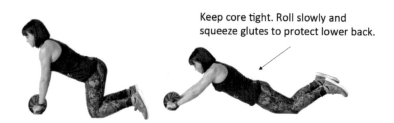

Keep core tight. Roll slowly and squeeze glutes to protect lower back.

C Reverse the motion and roll SLOWLY backwards, lifting knees up as you get closer to your feet, then stand and jump. Keep the wheel close to your hips.

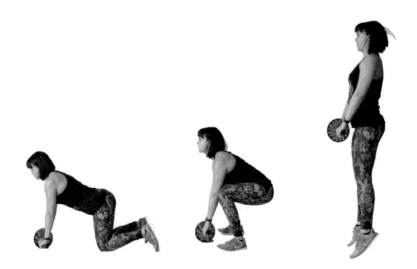

BURPEE VARIATION #97:

TIRE FLIP BURPEE

Equipment needed: Tractor tire. Weight varies, please plan accordingly for lifts. We like a lighter, mid-range for burpees that can be deadlifted vs. an athletic lift required for heavier tires.

A Start standing in front of the tire. Hinge from the hips and place hands wide with fingertips underneath the tire. Drive from your legs to extend through the hips. Your hips should help send the tire forward and upward with your body, use knee if needed (for heavier tires) to flip it all the way over. Keep tire close to body and quickly rotate hands when you flip it.

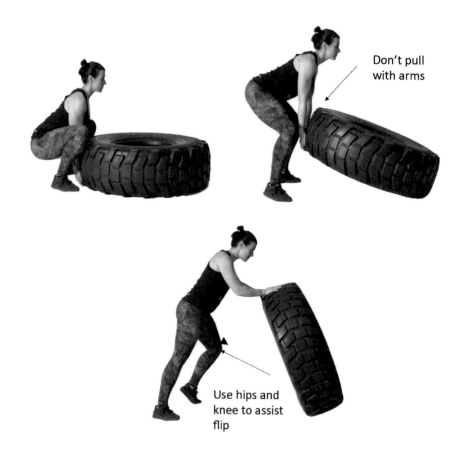

Don't pull with arms

Use hips and knee to assist flip

B Once the tire is flipped over, place hands on the edge of the tire and do a push-up. Bring feet back to hands and jump into the air in front of the tire.

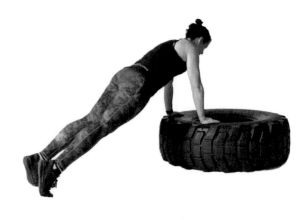

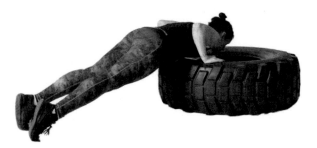

BURPEE VARIATION #98:

TIRE BURPEE

Equipment needed: Heavy tractor tire. Weight varies, please plan accordingly.

 Start standing in front of the tire. Jump on and off the tire. Place hands on the tire and do a push-up. Hop feet back to hands and jump up in front of the tire.

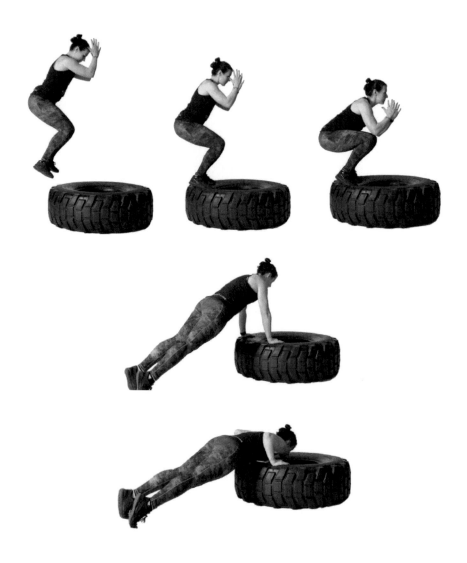

BURPEE VARIATION #99:

PULLING WEIGHT BURPEE

Equipment needed: Battle rope or other sturdy rope. Plate weight (we used 45 lb.– adjust up or down according to client fitness level). Attach rope to weight securely.

A Set weight 10-20 feet away from you depending on space and fitness level. Straddle rope in a 1/2 squat, and pull rope towards you hand over hand until it is directly in front of you.

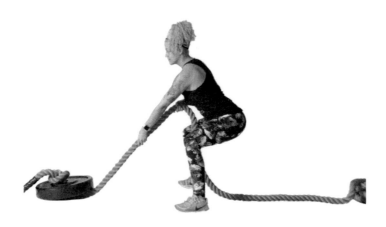

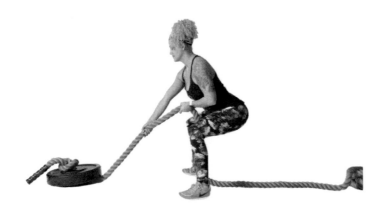

B Drop down and do a push-up while straddled over the rope. Finish the burpee with a jump. Land straddled. Reset and repeat

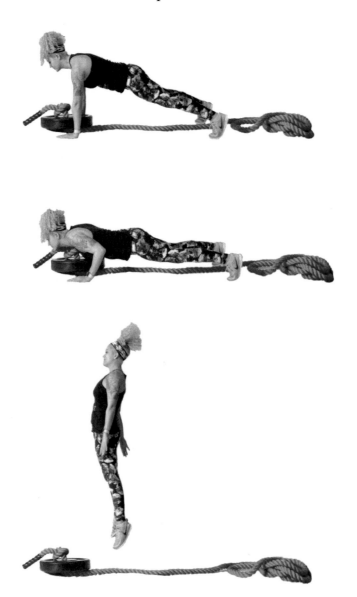

BURPEE VARIATION #100:

PUSHING WEIGHT BURPEE

Equipment needed: Plate weight (we used 45 lb.– adjust up or down according to client fitness level). Test floor surface for slideability.

A Start in plank with the weight between hands. Bend arms and crouch down (as much or little as needed) as you push the weight forward a little with one arm. Return to plank, hop feet back to hands and jump up. Return to plank and slide weight forward with the other arm. Repeat jump to finish the burpee.

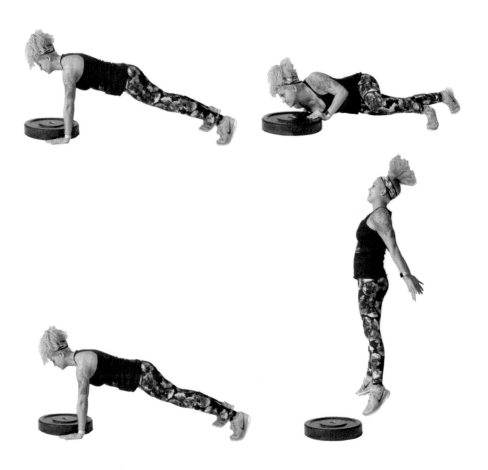

TRAINER'S TIP: Advanced burpee. Add a push-up before jumping up to add difficulty. Set a distance as a goal as space allows or just do 2 reps.

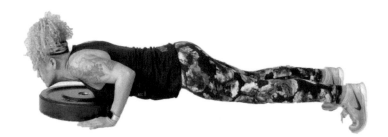

BONUS: BURPEE CHALLENGES

30 DAY BURPEE CHALLENGE GFD1

Start with 7 different burpees. One for each day of the week. We chose 7 for you. You can change those 7 so this challenge is different every time you decide to do it!

Monday: Regular burpees

Tuesday: Broad jump burpees

Wednesday: Hit the Deck Burpee

Thursday: Grasshopper Burpees

Friday: Corn on the Cob Burpees

Sat: Donkey Kick Burpees

Sun: Zen Burpees

Do the following reps of each burpee according to the week:

Week 1: 10 Reps a day

Week 2: 20 Reps a day

Week 3: 30 Reps a day

Week 4: 40 Reps a day

Week 5: 50 Reps a day

This is an advanced set up. Add a rest day if desired, and lower the reps for newer clients.

30 DAY BURPEE CHALLENGE GFD2

Start with 7 different burpees. One for each day of the week. We chose 7 for you. Rotate the 7 each week so you are doing different reps of the different burpees each week. You can change those 7 so this challenge is different every time you decide to do it!

Do the following reps of each burpee according to the week:

Week 1: 10 Reps a day as follows:

Monday: Regular burpees

Tuesday: Star Jump Burpees

Wednesday: Caterpillar Burpees

Thursday: Sit Thru Burpees

Friday: Elevator Burpees

Sat: Snowboarding Style Burpees

Sun: Zen Burpees

Week 2: 20 Reps a day as follows:

Monday: Star Jump Burpees

Tuesday: Sit Thru Burpees

Wednesday: Elevator Burpees

Thursday: Snowboarding Style Burpees

Friday: Regular Burpees

Week 3: 30 Reps a day as follows:

Monday: Zen Burpees

Tuesday: Elevator Burpees

Wednesday: Star Jump Burpees

Thursday: Regular Burpees

Friday: Sit Thru Burpees

Sat: Caterpillar Burpees

Sun: Snowboarding Style Burpees

Week 4: 40 Reps a day as follows:

Monday: Star Jump Burpees

Tuesday: Sit Thru Burpees

Wednesday: Elevator Burpees

Thursday: Snowboarding Style Burpees

Friday: Regular Burpees

Sat: Zen Burpees

Sun: Caterpillar Burpees

Week 5: 50 Reps a day as follows:

Monday: Sit Thru Burpees

Tuesday: Caterpillar Burpees

Wednesday: Snowboarding Style Burpees

Thursday: Elevator Burpees

Friday: Zen Burpees

Sat: Star Jump Burpees

Sun: Regular Burpees

This is an advanced set up. Add a rest day if desired, and lower the reps for newer clients.

30 DAY BURPEE CHALLENGE GFD3

This is a 100 Burpee end goal challenge. It incorporates rest days which allows for most clients to follow. Choose one burpee per week (5 burpees) 1 burpee for the whole month, or one burpee per day. Modify as needed.

Day 1: 5 Burpees	Day 11: 35 Burpees	Day 21: 65 Burpees
Day 2: 10 Burpees	Day 12: 40 Burpees	Day 22: 70 Burpees
Day 3: 15 Burpees	Day 13: 45 Burpees	Day 23: 75 Burpees
Day 4: 20 Burpees	Day 14: 50 burpees	Day 24: 80 Burpees
Day 5: REST	Day 15: REST	Day 25: REST
Day 6: 20 Burpees	Day 16: 50 Burpees	Day 26: 80 Burpees
Day 7: 25 Burpees	Day 17: 55 Burpees	Day 27: 85 Burpees
Day 8: 30 Burpees	Day 18: 60 Burpees	Day 28: 90 Burpees
Day 9: 35 Burpees	Day 19: 65 Burpees	Day 29: 95 Burpees
Day 10: REST	Day 20: REST	Day 30: 100 Burpees

30 DAY BURPEE CHALLENGE GFD4

This is a 120 Burpee end goal challenge. Choose one burpee per week, one burpee for the whole month, or one burpee per day. Modify as needed.

Day 1: 5 Burpees	Day 11: 45 Burpees	Day 21: REST
Day 2: 10 Burpees	Day 12: 50 Burpees	Day 22: 80 Burpees
Day 3: 15 Burpees	Day 13: 55 Burpees	Day 23: 85 Burpees
Day 4: 20 Burpees	Day 14: REST	Day 24: 90 Burpees
Day 5: 25 Burpees	Day 15: 55 Burpees	Day 25: 95 Burpees
Day 6: 30 Burpees	Day 16: 60 Burpees	Day 26: 100 Burpees
Day 7: REST	Day 17: 65 Burpees	Day 27: 105 Burpees
Day 8: 30 Burpees	Day 18: 70 Burpees	Day 28: 110 Burpees
Day 9: 35 Burpees	Day 19: 75 Burpees	Day 29: 115 Burpees
Day 10: 40 Burpees	Day 20: 80 Burpees	Day 30: 120 Burpees

7 DAY BURPEE CHALLENGE GFD5
THE GO TO 7 DAY TRAVEL
BURPEE CHALLENGE

Traveling? NO excuse. These bodyweight burpees can be done in your hotel room, on the beach, etc. Use common sense and don't get hurt!

Each # of reps can be reduced or increased depending on fitness level. Each Burpee can be changed to your liking and ability. Enjoy your travel! Warm up properly.

Day 1:

20 Regular Burpees

20 Crow Pose Burpees

20 Dirty Double Jack Burpees

Day 2:

20 Regular Burpees

20 Single Leg Burpees

20 Half Burpees

Day 3:

25 Regular Burpees

25 Zen Burpees

25 Mountain Climber Burpees

Day 4 or Rest:

25 Regular Burpees

25 Grasshopper Burpees

25 Hip Dip Burpees

Day 5:

30 Regular Burpees

30 Side Sprawl Burpees

30 T-Push-up Burpees

Day 6:

30 Regular Burpees

30 Sprinting Burpees

30 Deadman Burpees

Day 7 or Rest:

20 Regular Burpees

20 Doggie Burpees

20 Twisted Burpees

BURPEE FINISHERS

Add these to the end of your workout as a burner or a separate challenge. Change the burpees and reps according to ability and fitness level. Rest 1-3 minutes between rounds.

100 Rep Burpee Workout

Do 5 reps of each of these 5 burpees for 4 rounds:

Tuck Jump Burpee

Broad Jump Burpee

Crow Pose Burpee

Caterpillar Burpee

Half Burpee

500 Rep Burpee Workout

Do 10 reps of each of these 5 burpees for 10 rounds:

Dirty Double Plank Jack Burpee

Inchworm Burpee

Skater Hop Burpee

Single Leg Push-up Burpee (5 each side)

Bird Dog Burpee (5 each side)

1000 Rep Burpee Workout

Do 10 reps of each of these 10 burpees for 10 rounds:

Ninja Burpee

Snowboarding Style Burpee

Shoulder Tap Burpee

T-Push up Burpee (5 each side)

Staggered Jump Burpee (5 each side)

Plank Jack Burpee

Mountain Climber Burpee

One Arm Burpee

Bulldog Burpee

Squat Burpee

Made in the USA
Columbia, SC
28 February 2019